Current Challenges and Advances in Skin Repair and Regeneration

Current Challenges and Advances in Skin Repair and Regeneration

Guest Editor

Giovanni Salzano

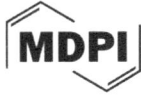

Basel • Beijing • Wuhan • Barcelona • Belgrade • Novi Sad • Cluj • Manchester

Guest Editor
Giovanni Salzano
Department of Reproductive
and Odontostomatological
Neurosciences
University of Naples
Federico II
Naples
Italy

Editorial Office
MDPI AG
Grosspeteranlage 5
4052 Basel, Switzerland

This is a reprint of the Special Issue, published open access by the journal *Journal of Clinical Medicine* (ISSN 2077-0383), freely accessible at: https://www.mdpi.com/journal/jcm/special_issues/Skin_Repair_Regeneration.

For citation purposes, cite each article independently as indicated on the article page online and as indicated below:

Lastname, A.A.; Lastname, B.B. Article Title. *Journal Name* **Year**, *Volume Number*, Page Range.

ISBN 978-3-7258-4101-1 (Hbk)
ISBN 978-3-7258-4102-8 (PDF)
https://doi.org/10.3390/books978-3-7258-4102-8

© 2025 by the authors. Articles in this book are Open Access and distributed under the Creative Commons Attribution (CC BY) license. The book as a whole is distributed by MDPI under the terms and conditions of the Creative Commons Attribution-NonCommercial-NoDerivs (CC BY-NC-ND) license (https://creativecommons.org/licenses/by-nc-nd/4.0/).

Contents

Youn Hwan Kim, Hyung Sup Shim, Jihye Lee and Sang Wha Kim
A Prospective Randomized Controlled Multicenter Clinical Trial Comparing Paste-Type
Acellular Dermal Matrix to Standard Care for the Treatment of Chronic Wounds
Reprinted from: *J. Clin. Med.* **2022**, *11*, 2203, https://doi.org/10.3390/jcm11082203 1

Tomasz Korzeniowski, Paulina Mertowska, Sebastian Mertowski, Martyna Podgajna,
Ewelina Grywalska, Jerzy Strużyna and Kamil Torres
The Role of the Immune System in Pediatric Burns: A Systematic Review
Reprinted from: *J. Clin. Med.* **2022**, *11*, 2262, https://doi.org/10.3390/jcm11082262 12

Raffaele Russo, Albino Carrizzo, Alfonso Barbato, Barbara Rosa Rasile, Paola Pentangelo,
Alessandra Ceccaroni, et al.
Clinical Evaluation of the Efficacy and Tolerability of Rigenase® and Polyhexanide
(Fitostimoline® Plus) vs. Hyaluronic Acid and Silver Sulfadiazine (Connettivina® Bio Plus) for
the Treatment of Acute Skin Wounds: A Randomized Trial
Reprinted from: *J. Clin. Med.* **2022**, *11*, 2518, https://doi.org/10.3390/jcm11092518 26

Byung Woo Yoo, Seungyoon Oh, Junekyu Kim, Kap Sung Oh, Hyun Woo Shin and
Kyu Nam Kim
Modified Mini-Keystone Flaps for Coverage of Tiny Volar Pulp Defects of the Fingertips in
Cases with Missing Amputation Skin Stumps: A Retrospective Study
Reprinted from: *J. Clin. Med.* **2022**, *11*, 3394, https://doi.org/10.3390/jcm11123394 37

Dinko Martinovic, Slaven Lupi-Ferandin, Daria Tokic, Mislav Usljebrka, Andrija Rados,
Ante Pojatina, et al.
Objective Skin Quality Assessment after Reconstructive Procedures for Facial Skin Defects
Reprinted from: *J. Clin. Med.* **2022**, *11*, 4471, https://doi.org/10.3390/jcm11154471 48

Tomasz Korzeniowski, Ewelina Grywalska, Jerzy Strużyna, Magdalena Bugaj-Tobiasz,
Agnieszka Surowiecka, Izabela Korona-Głowniak, et al.
Preliminary Single-Center Experience of Bromelain-Based Eschar Removal in Children with
Mixed Deep Dermal and Full Thickness Burns
Reprinted from: *J. Clin. Med.* **2022**, *11*, 4800, https://doi.org/10.3390/jcm11164800 60

Antonio Arena, Umberto Committeri, Fabio Maglitto, Giovanni Salzano,
Giovanni Dell'Aversana Orabona, Luigi Angelo Vaira, et al.
Three Different Types of Fat Grafting for Facial Systemic Sclerosis: A Case Series
Reprinted from: *J. Clin. Med.* **2022**, *11*, 5489, https://doi.org/10.3390/jcm11185489 71

Anis Anis, Ahmed Sharshar, Saber El Hanbally and Awad A. Shehata
Histopathological Evaluation of the Healing Process of Standardized Skin Burns in Rabbits:
Assessment of a Natural Product with Honey and Essential Oils
Reprinted from: *J. Clin. Med.* **2022**, *11*, 6417, https://doi.org/10.3390/jcm11216417 78

Hanna Luze, Ives Bernardelli de Mattos, Sebastian Philipp Nischwitz, Martin Funk,
Alexandru Cristian Tuca and Lars-Peter Kamolz
The Impact of Antiseptic-Loaded Bacterial Nanocellulose on Different Biofilms—An Effective
Treatment for Chronic Wounds?
Reprinted from: *J. Clin. Med.* **2022**, *11*, 6634, https://doi.org/10.3390/jcm11226634 90

**Giovanni Salzano, Francesco Maffia, Luigi Angelo Vaira, Umberto Committeri,
Chiara Copelli, Fabio Maglitto, et al.**
Locoregional Flaps for the Reconstruction of Midface Skin Defects: A Collection of Key Surgical Techniques
Reprinted from: *J. Clin. Med.* **2023**, *12*, 3700, https://doi.org/10.3390/jcm12113700 . . . . **104**

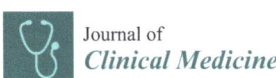

Article

A Prospective Randomized Controlled Multicenter Clinical Trial Comparing Paste-Type Acellular Dermal Matrix to Standard Care for the Treatment of Chronic Wounds

Youn Hwan Kim [1,†], Hyung Sup Shim [2,†], Jihye Lee [3] and Sang Wha Kim [4,*]

1. Department of Plastic and Reconstructive Surgery, College of Medicine, Hanyang University, Seoul 04763, Korea; younhwank@daum.net
2. Department of Plastic and Reconstructive Surgery, College of Medicine, The Catholic University of Korea, St. Vincent's Hospital, Seoul 06591, Korea; shrapshim@catholic.ac.kr
3. CG Bio, Seoul 04349, Korea; jhlee2818@cgbio.co.kr
4. Department of Plastic and Reconstructive Surgery, College of Medicine, Seoul National University, Seoul National University Hospital, Seoul 03080, Korea
* Correspondence: sw1215@snu.ac.kr; Tel.: +82-2-2072-2375; Fax: +82-2-3675-7792
† These authors contributed equally to this work.

Abstract: The treatment of chronic wounds remains challenging. Acellular dermal matrix (ADM) has been shown to be effective for various types of wound healing. This study was designed to compare the wound size reduction rate after 12 weeks between patients receiving paste-type ADM and standard wound care. Patients over 19 years old with chronic wounds, deeper than full-thickness skin defects, more than 4 cm^2 in size that did not heal over the 3 weeks before the study were included. After a screening period of 7 days, patients were randomized to receive either paste-type ADM or standard wound care. The wound status was evaluated at baseline, 1, 2, 4, 8, and 12 weeks. A total of 86 patients were enrolled in this study. The wounds continuously and constantly reduced in size from week 1, and the reduction rate was significantly greater in the study group from week 2 until the end (week 12). In the study group, wound healing was achieved in 29 of 38 wounds (76.3%). Paste-type ADM might be a useful option for wound healing and can be applied safely and efficiently for advanced wound care.

Keywords: acellular dermis; wound healing; ulcer

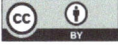

1. Introduction

Wound healing progresses systematically through inflammation, proliferation, and remodeling phases [1,2]. Interference in this well-coordinated process, especially in the inflammatory stage, leads to chronic non-healing wounds [2]. Chronic wounds often occur in patients with comorbidities such as diabetes, vascular problems (including arterial disease and venous ulcers), or chronic inflammation (such as osteomyelitis, autoimmune disease, and radiation ulcers) [3–6]. It is estimated that 1–2% of the population of developed countries experience chronic wounds [5], which not only affect quality of life but also increase healthcare costs [3,7,8].

The treatment of chronic wounds remains challenging. When these wounds are non-responsive to conventional wound management modalities, advanced wound care materials, including cultured autologous material, allogenic materials, and bioengineered products, are required to accelerate wound healing [3,9–12].

Acellular dermal matrix (ADM) is a biomaterial derived from autologous and allogenic tissues that undergoes processing to remove cells, while still retaining the bioactive dermal matrix, consisting of collagen, elastin, and fibronectin [2–4,7]. ADM has been used widely in various applications as a dermal replacement, including for the head and neck, breast, abdominal wall, and extremity reconstruction, and has also been shown to be effective for tissue regeneration and wound healing [2–4,7,12–14].

Although ADM is commonly used in sheet form, paste-type ADM manufactured by crushing and micronizing allograft material derived from donated human skin has recently been introduced. This transformation makes it is easy to handle and paste-type ADM can be applied to various types of wounds, including external, ulcerative and irregularly shaped tunneling wounds [7,12–15]. Previous studies have demonstrated the efficacy of sheet-type ADM as a dermal substitute for various types of wound reconstruction [2,4]. Other studies have reported the outcomes of ADM therapy for chronic wounds, such as diabetic foot ulcers [10–12,16,17]. However, few studies have used paste-type ADM, and most were not randomized controlled studies.

The primary objective of this study was to compare the wound size reduction rate after 12 weeks between patients receiving ADM therapy and standard wound care. The secondary objectives were to compare the complete wound healing rate, the epithelization rate, granulation tissue formation, and safety.

2. Materials and Methods

This was a 12-week prospective randomized controlled multicenter clinical trial conducted to determine the efficacy and safety of paste-type ADM therapy. This study was approved by the institutional review boards of Seoul National University (1704-063-845), Hanyang University (2017-01-061), and the Catholic University of Korea (VC17DNSI0079). All participants provided written informed consent for the publication of the case details, including images. The study was registered at ClinicalTrials.gov (NCT04019639). All of the data were analyzed anonymously and in accordance with the principles of the 1975 Declaration of Helsinki (revised in 2008).

Two products were used in this study: CG-PASTE (CG Bio Co., Ltd., Seoul, Korea) and Easyfoam (CG Bio Co., Ltd., Seoul, Korea). CG-PASTE is a paste-type micronized acellular dermal matrix that is currently used safely in clinical practice; it has been approved as a medical device applicable to open wounds except for third-degree burns. Easyfoam is a wound dressing applied to wounds with exudates and protects wounds by maintaining a moist environment on the wound.

Each patient was screened for eligibility, including a complete medical history, physical examination, and full assessment of the wound, based on the inclusion and exclusion criteria shown in Table 1.

Table 1. Inclusion and exclusion criteria.

Inclusion Criteria	Exclusion Criteria
• Patients > 19 years old • Full-thickness skin defects to bone exposure wounds • Wounds measuring > 4 cm2 • Wounds failing to heal following a minimum of 3 weeks of conservative care prior to the study • Wounds without uncontrolled infection • HbA1c ≤ 12% within the previous 3 months • Serum creatinine ≤ 3.0 mg/dL	• Superficial or partial thickness skin defects • Undermining or tunneling wounds • Wounds with uncontrolled infection • HbA1c > 12% within the previous 3 months • Serum creatinine > 3.0 mg/dL • Treatment with other medical devices or topical growth factors within the previous 30 days

Patients > 19 years old, with chronic wounds with the wound depth ranging from full-thickness skin to bone exposure measuring more than 4 cm^2 and failing to heal during a minimum of 3 weeks before the study [9,10,15], were eligible for inclusion.

The exclusion criteria were superficial or partial-thickness skin defects, undermining or tunneling wounds for which it was difficult to measure the wound depth, and uncontrolled infection, including osteomyelitis. Patients with poor metabolic control (HgA1c > 12% within the previous 3 months), a serum creatinine level > 3.0 mg/dL, treatment with other medical devices or topical growth factors that can influence wound healing within the previous 30 days were excluded.

Patients were evaluated during a screening period up to 7 days before baseline surgical debridement and treatment. All patients underwent debridement until healthy, viable tissue was visible in the wounds. After the surgical preparation of the wound site, patients were randomized into either the experimental group (paste-type ADM and conventional dressing) or control group (conventional dressing) using sequentially numbered, opaque, sealed envelopes to avoid selection bias.

Wounds were assessed at 0 (baseline, after initial surgical preparation of wound site), 1, 2, 4, 8, and 12 weeks after randomization, and upon study exit or withdrawal. Photographs of the wounds were taken at a distance of 30 cm. A centimeter scale was placed adjacent to the wound. Wound size, granulation tissue formation, epithelization, complete healing status, and adverse events were recorded at each follow-up visit.

For patients assigned to the experimental group, paste-type ADM (CGPaste) was placed on the wound bed to cover the entire wound surface, and then covered with polyurethane foam (EasyFoam). It was applied at 0, 1, 2, and 4 weeks after the initial surgical preparation of the wound. For patients in the control group, wounds were covered with conventional dressing using polyurethane foam only.

The main outcome was wound size reduction over the 12-week follow-up period. Secondary outcomes were the achievement of complete healing (defined as an epithelized wound with no raw surface and no requirement for additional wound management), time to complete healing, and granulation tissue formation during the follow-up period. Wound granulation and epithelialization were evaluated by using photographs of the wounds taken under similar conditions (distance, brightness, etc.). The evaluation of photographs was performed by two independent evaluators who are experts in the plastic surgery department. Granulation tissue formation was evaluated as the percentage of the wound surface that was covered with bright-red healthy granulation tissue. The granulation rate was defined as the percentage of patients who achieved over 75% granulation. Epithelialization is defined as the wound covered with an epithelial surface. The epithelialization rate was calculated as the percentage of patients who achieved epithelization. Adverse events, including wound infection or any complications, were also evaluated.

Statistical Analysis

Categorical variables were analyzed using contingency tables (Chi-square) and continuous variables were analyzed using either the independent *t*-test or Mann–Whitney test, depending on whether the data met the criteria for parametric analysis. The times to healing and granulation were compared between the two treatment arms using the log-rank test. A statistical analysis was performed using GraphPad Prism for Windows (version 5; GraphPad Software Inc., San Diego, CA, USA), and a two-sided $p < 0.05$ was taken to indicate statistical significance.

3. Results

A flow chart of study enrollment and participation through the clinical trial is shown in Figure 1.

According to the literature, the chronic wound area of the control group after 12 weeks was expected to decrease by about 92.3% compared to the baseline [18], and that of the test group' was expected to decrease by about 98% [19]. Therefore, in this study, it was assumed that reasonable clinical improvement was reached when the difference between the groups in wound area reduction rate was 6% or more (80% power and 5% significance level). The sample size for this clinical trial was calculated as 84 patients (42 patients per group), taking into consideration a 15% drop-out rate.

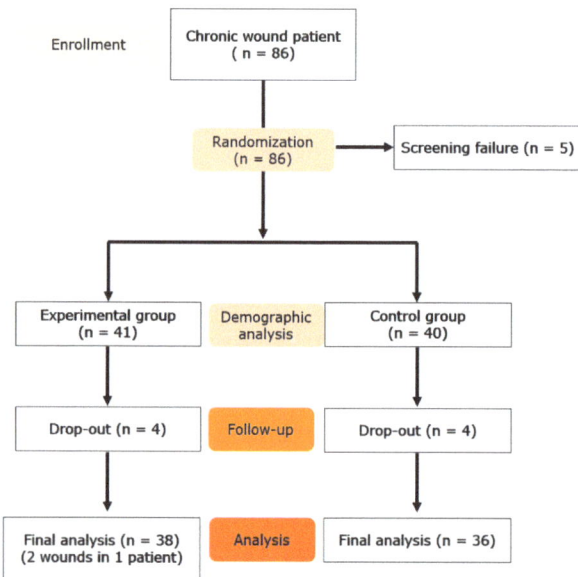

Figure 1. Flow of study enrollment and participation.

Of the 86 patients enrolled in the study, five were considered screening failures. The remaining 81 patients were randomized into two treatment groups, with 41 patients (42 wounds) receiving paste-type ADM (study group) and 40 (40 wounds) receiving standard care (control group). Eight patients (four in the study group and four in the control group) did not complete the clinical trial.

Table 2 shows a comparison of demographic characteristics, including the initial wound size between the two groups upon enrollment. The two groups were comparable in terms of age, sex, and comorbidities (including diabetes, hypertension, autoimmune disease, and vascular disease). The baseline wound size was also not significantly different between the groups.

The wound size reductions at the evaluation points in both treatment groups are presented in Table 3. The wounds showed a continuous and relatively constant reduction from week 1 in the study group and week 4 in the control group (Figure 2). There was a significant difference in the wound area reduction rate between the groups from week 2 to the study endpoint (week 12).

The percentage of granulation tissue in the wound (Figure 3), as well as the wound epithelization rate (Figure 4), showed substantial increases over time. The differences between the groups were clinically significant for both parameters ($p = 0.0006$ and $p = 0.0016$, respectively).

Wound healing was defined as complete epithelization without a raw surface. Figure 5 shows the percentage of wounds that healed completely over the course of treatment. In the study group, 29 of 38 wounds (76.32%) were healed by 12 weeks, compared to only 11 of 36 (30.56%) in the control group ($p = 0.001$).

No adverse events were noted during treatment.

Table 2. Demographic characteristics.

		Experimental Group (N = 41)	Control Group (N = 40)	p-Value
Age (Year)	Mean ± SD	58.71 ± 16.33	63.63 ± 13.47	0.1436
Sex	Male, N(%)	23 (56.1)	19 (47.5)	0.4415
	Female, N(%)	18 (43.9)	21 (52.5)	
Smoking	No, N (%)	34 (82.9)	28 (70.0)	0.1735
	Yes, N (%)	7 (17.1)	12 (30.0)	
Alcohol consumption	No, N (%)	33 (80.5)	30 (75.0)	0.5541
	Yes, N (%)	8 (19.5)	10 (25.0)	
Diabetes	No, N (%)	28 (68.3)	24 (60.0)	0.4388
	Yes, N (%)	13 (31.7)	16 (40.0)	
Hypertension	No, N (%)	31 (75.6)	24 (60.0)	0.1351
	Yes, N (%)	10 (24.4)	16 (40.0)	
Hemodialysis	No, N (%)	37 (90.2)	38 (95.0)	0.4131
	Yes, N (%)	4 (9.8)	2 (5.0)	
Vascular disorder	No, N (%)	36 (87.8)	36 (90.0)	0.7543
	Yes, N (%)	5 (12.2)	4 (10.0)	
Wound area (cm^2)	Mean ± SD	18.01 ± 10.62	19.10 ± 15.37	0.7108

Table 3. Wound area reduction.

	Experimental Group	p-Value (vs. Baseline)		Control Group	p-Value (vs. Baseline)	p-Value (Ctrl vs. Exp.)
Baseline (n = 41)	18.01 ± 10.62	-	Baseline (n = 40)	19.10 ± 15.37	-	0.7108
Week 0 (n = 38)	17.57 ± 10.73	0.8544	Week 0 (n = 36)	19.86 ± 15.89	0.8328	0.4677
Week 1 (n = 37)	13.00 ± 9.63	* 0.0319	Week 1 (n = 36)	18.40 ± 14.89	0.8411	0.0692
Week 2 (n = 38)	8.56 ± 6.31	* <0.0001	Week 2 (n = 36)	16.65 ± 12.93	0.4572	* 0.0009
Week 4 (n = 38)	5.05 ± 5.38	* <0.0001	Week 4 (n = 36)	11.96 ± 9.46	* 0.01	* 0.0002
Week 8 (n = 38)	1.92 ± 3.96	* <0.0001	Week 8 (n = 36)	7.69 ± 7.43	* 0.0001	* 0.0001
Week 12 (n = 38)	0.90 ± 2.77	* <0.0001	Week 12 (n = 36)	5.69 ± 5.58	* <0.0001	* <0.0001

* indicates statistical significance ($p < 0.05$).

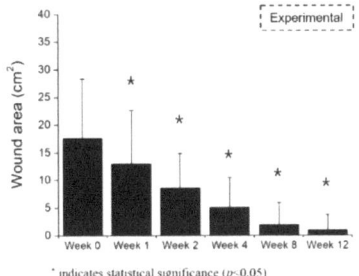
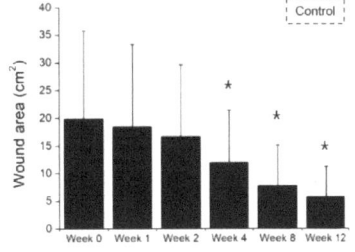

Figure 2. Wound area reduction by week.

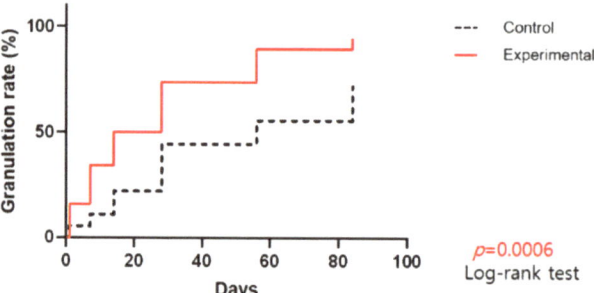

Figure 3. Percentage of granulation tissue in the wound by day.

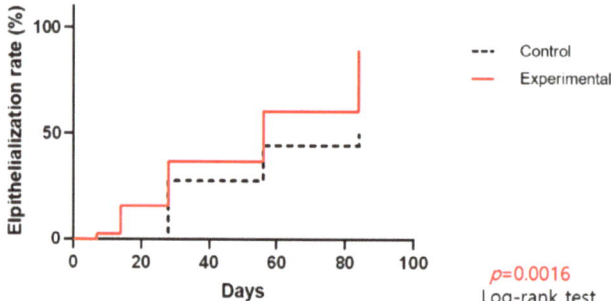

Figure 4. Wound epithelization rate by day.

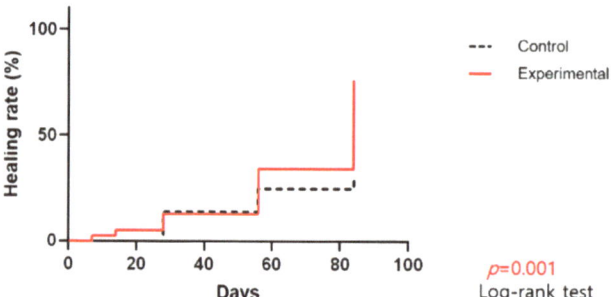

Figure 5. Percentage of wounds completely healed throughout the course of treatment.

3.1. Case 1

A 27-year-old female patient presented with a third-degree contact burn on her lower left leg. After debridement, the wound measured 6.0 × 4 cm (Figure 6). We applied 2 cc of paste-type ADM and covered the wound with polyurethane foam dressing. After 4 weeks, the wound size had reduced by approximately 50%, and it had healed almost completely after week 8, but the epithelialized wound appeared "scratched" due to trauma. Complete healing was observed by week 12.

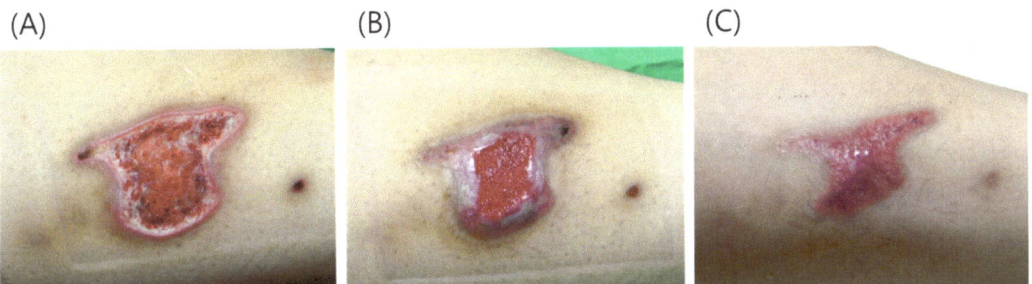

Figure 6. (**A**) A 27-year-old female patient presented with a third-degree contact burn on her lower left leg. (**B**) After 4 weeks, the wound size had reduced by approximately 50%. (**C**) At week 12, the wound had healed completely.

3.2. Case 2

An 81-year-old male patient presented with an open wound on his lower left leg due to trauma. The patient was treated at a local clinic for over 1 month, but the wound did not heal. A 5 × 4 cm skin defect was observed after debridement (Figure 7). We applied 2 cc of paste-type ADM with a polyurethane foam dressing. Paste-type ADM was reapplied at 1, 2, and 4 weeks. At week 8 after initial treatment, the wound size had reduced to 1.5 × 2 cm. After 12 weeks, the wound had healed completely. No contracture deformity was observed and a good esthetic outcome was achieved.

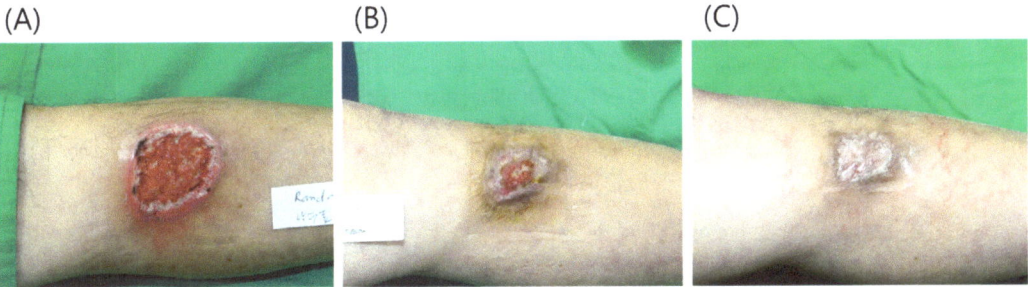

Figure 7. (**A**) A 52-year-old male patient presented with a 5 × 4 cm skin defect on his lower left leg. (**B**) At 8 weeks after initial treatment, the wound size had reduced to 1.5 × 2 cm. (**C**) At 12 weeks, the wound was completely healed without contracture deformity.

3.3. Case 3

A 77-year-old male patient presented with a diabetic foot ulcer in the right lateral malleolus region. A rotation flap was applied from the foot dorsum and skin grafting was performed at the donor site. However, the flap was necrotized and the skin graft only partially took. After debridement, an open wound measuring about 5 × 3 cm was observed in the lateral malleolus region and on the foot (Figure 8). After the application of paste-type ADM at weeks 0, 1, and 2, the wound on the foot healed almost completely and the wound on the lateral malleolus was covered with healthy granulation tissue. The wound gradually reduced in size, and showed complete healing by week 12.

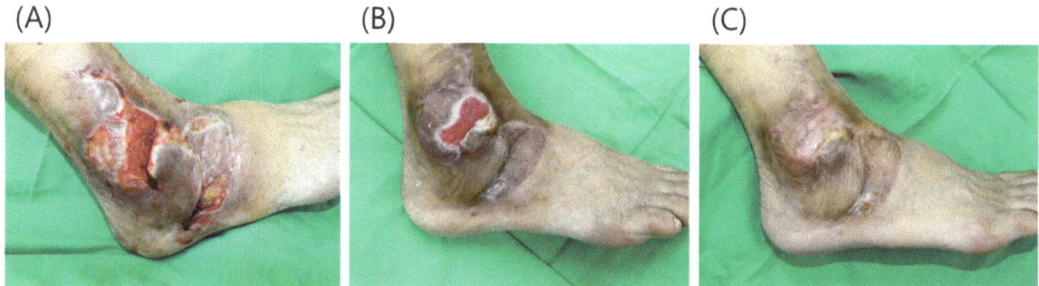

Figure 8. (**A**) A 65-year-old male patient presented with a diabetic foot ulcer. (**B**) After 4 weeks, the wound on the foot had healed almost completely and the wound at the lateral malleolus was covered with healthy granulation tissue. (**C**) At week 12, the wound had healed completely without discomfort in the foot or ankle; normal function also returned.

The patient was satisfied that the wound had healed completely without surgery, with no discomfort in the foot or ankle and normal function.

4. Discussion

Wound healing is a well-coordinated process involving interactions of cells with the microenvironment. The extracellular matrix (ECM) is one of the key elements in wound healing, providing structural support as the largest component of the dermal layer [2,15] and also promoting effective wound healing by providing signaling proteins for cell adhesion and signaling [10,20–22]. As the ECM is often dysfunctional or insufficient in chronic wounds, it is challenging to promote wound healing. Efforts have been made to replace the damaged ECM or restore its function to stimulate wound healing [2,3]. The application of ADM has been applied as an alternative for the ECM in chronic wounds [15,23,24].

The use of ADM provides several advantages. First, the ADM undergone processing to remove cellular components, which makes it immunologically inert [3,4,7,12]. Second, the ADM scaffold comprised of collagen, elastin, and fibronectin provides a favorable microenvironment for cellular proliferation and vascularization [7,12,25]. Third, by retaining the function of the ECM in cell adhesion and cell signaling, ADM promotes fibroblast attachment, attracts vascular endothelial cells, and helps growth factors [15,26–28]. These properties allow the initiation of self-regeneration processes of wound healing in chronic non-healing wounds [14,29]. Interactions between the surrounding tissue and ADM could result in wound healing by re-epithelialization or granulation tissue formation [14].

This study used paste-type ADM, which is crushed, micronized, and packed in a syringe, and can therefore be applied more easily than sheet-type ADM. Most of the participants in this study were enrolled on an outpatient basis. In addition, it can be applied to complicated wounds, including deep wounds, cavitary wounds, undermining and tunneling wounds, wounds with dead space, etc. [7,30,31]. Therefore, paste-type ADM is particularly useful for sores and diabetic ulcers, where it can be adjusted to maximize contact with irregular surfaces.

The clinical efficacy of a paste-type ADM for various wounds has recently been studied in animal experiments and clinical trials. However, there has been little progress in clinical studies and most such reports to date have been case studies. Paste-type ADM has shown comparable effectiveness for wound healing to subcutaneous injection in rat models [14]. Several authors have reported the clinical efficacy of the ADM application for wound coverage. Early retrospective case studies suggested that ADM may promote wound healing without surgery [7,32]. Jeon and Kim performed a retrospective study with application of ADM to chronic wounds, and wound healing was achieved in 2.4 weeks on average in five out of seven cases [30]. Ahn et al. performed a prospective clinical trial of 20 patients using paste-type ADM in conjunction with negative pressure wound therapy (NPWT), achieving a wound area reduction rate of 59.1% after 4 weeks [15]. In a single-center randomized controlled trial, Brigido compared the application of human ADM to conventional methods using gauze dressing in uninfected wounds of the lower extremities and showed that 12 of 14 patients (85.7%) in the ADM group achieved complete healing after the 16 weeks of treatment, in comparison to only 4 of 14 patients (28.7%) in the control group [7]. Hahn et al. performed a prospective randomized pilot study of micronized human ADM in 30 patients with diabetic foot ulcers, comparing the application of ADM to conventional NPWT, and reported that 93.3% of patients in the experimental group and 85.7% in the conventional therapy group achieved complete wound healing during the 6-month follow-up [31].

The results of this prospective randomized multicenter study indicated that chronic wounds treated with ADM have a higher probability of healing compared to those treated with conventional management. This study had two main goals. The first was to compare the wound size reduction rate after 12 weeks between patients receiving paste-type ADM and standard wound care, and the second was to compare the epithelization rate, growth of granulation tissue, complete wound healing rate, and safety between treatment groups. Immediately after surgical preparation and the application of ADM, the wound size continuously and constantly reduced from week 1, and from week 2, the wound size reduction was significantly greater in the study group until the end (week 12). Furthermore, granulation tissue formation was observed in 36 of 38 wounds (94.7%) in the study group compared to 26 of 36 wounds (72.2%) in the control group, while full epithelization was observed in 34 of 38 wounds (89.5%) in the study group and 18 of 36 wounds (50%) in the control group. Consequently, wound healing was achieved in 29 of 38 wounds (76.3%) in the study group compared to 11 of 36 wounds (30.6%) in the control group. In addition, no adverse events were noted during treatment.

Although debridement is not the standard of care for wound management, it was performed in this study to ensure that the two treatment groups were treated equally, and to promote wound healing while minimizing differences by wound type. The failure of wound healing is often caused by a prolonged inflammatory phase or poor vascularization. Debridement reduces the bacterial burden, removes biofilms and necrotic tissue, ensures viable cells at the wound edges, and helps prepare the wound bed before wound management. We assumed that the appropriate preparation of the wound bed improved the wound healing process in both treatment groups, resulting in complete wound healing in 40 of 74 wounds. There were no adverse events during treatment, including infection, indicating that the process was performed carefully in a sterile environment, and that the paste-type ADM infection rate is low such that it can be used safely.

The strengths of this study include the prospective randomized controlled design and involvement of multiple centers. Although 12 weeks is a common endpoint in wound studies, a longer follow-up would have been beneficial. In addition, there were no significant differences in demographic characteristics, including initial wound size, between the treatment groups, such that the outcomes reflected only the effects of the different treatments. The inclusion criterion was chronic non-healing wounds, with a depth from full-thickness skin defects to bone exposure, and a size measuring more than 4 cm^2 that failed to heal during a minimum of 3 weeks of conservative care before the study. As various factors can lead to chronic wounds, it is difficult to characterize a wound only according to location or type. Therefore, wound depth, size, and duration were considered in this study.

Regarding study limitations, paste-type ADM application was applied with polyurethane foam dressing in all cases. There may be differences in the effects of ADM according to the dressing material used at the same time. In addition, paste-type ADM was not compared to other types of conventional dressing, such as gauze or NPWT, or to other types of ADM.

This prospective randomized multicenter study showed that treatment of chronic wounds with ADM reduced wound size, increased the epithelization rate and granulation tissue formation, and achieved a higher rate of complete wound healing compared to conventional management. Therefore, paste-type ADM might be a useful option for wound healing and can be used safely and efficiently for advanced wound care.

Author Contributions: Data curation, H.S.S.; Investigation, Y.H.K.; Methodology, J.L.; Writing—original draft, S.W.K. All authors have read and agreed to the published version of the manuscript.

Funding: Korean Health Industry Development Institute: HI17C2295.

Institutional Review Board Statement: This study was approved by the institutional review boards of Seoul National University (1704-063-845), Hanyang University (2017-01-061), and the Catholic University of Korea (VC17DNSI0079). All participants provided written informed consent for the publication of the case details, including images. The study was registered at ClinicalTrials.gov (NCT04019639). All of the data were analyzed anonymously and in accordance with the principles of the 1975 Declaration of Helsinki (revised in 2008).

Informed Consent Statement: All participants provided written informed consent for the publication of the case details, including images.

Data Availability Statement: The data presented in this study are available on request from the corresponding author.

Acknowledgments: This research was supported by a grant of the Korea Health Technology R & D Project through the Korean Health Industry Development Institute (KHIDI), funded by the Ministry of Health & Welfare, Korea (grant number HI7C2295).

Conflicts of Interest: The authors declare no conflict of interest. The funders had no role in the design of the study; in the collection, analyses, or interpretation of data; in the writing of the manuscript, or in the decision to publish the results.

References

1. Werner, S.; Grose, R. Regulation of wound healing by growth factors and cytokines. *Physiol. Rev.* **2003**, *83*, 835–870. [CrossRef] [PubMed]
2. Kirsner, R.S.; Bohn, G.; Driver, V.R.; Mills, J.L.; Nanney, L.B.; Williams, M.L.; Wu, S.C. Human acellular dermal wound matrix: Evidence and experience. *Int. Wound J.* **2015**, *12*, 646–654. [CrossRef] [PubMed]
3. Schultz, G.S.; Davidson, J.M.; Kirsner, R.S.; Bornstein, P.; Herman, I.M. Dynamic reciprocity in the wound microenvironment. *Wound Repair Regen.* **2011**, *19*, 134–148. [CrossRef] [PubMed]
4. Hynes, R.O. Integrins: Bidirectional, allosteric signaling machines. *Cell* **2002**, *110*, 673–687. [CrossRef]
5. Berrier, A.L.; Yamada, K.M. Cell-matrix adhesion. *J. Cell Physiol.* **2007**, *213*, 565–573. [CrossRef]
6. Legate, K.R.; Wickstrom, S.A.; Fassler, R. Genetic and cell biological analysis of integrin outside-in signaling. *Genes Dev.* **2009**, *23*, 397–418. [CrossRef]
7. Cazzell, S.; Vayser, D.; Pham, H.; Walters, J.; Reyzelman, A.; Samsell, B.; Dorsch, K.; Moore, M. A randomized clinical trial of a human acellular dermal matrix demonstrated superior healing rates for chronic diabetic foot ulcers over conventional care and an active acellular dermal matrix comparator. *Wound Repair Regen.* **2017**, *25*, 483–497. [CrossRef]
8. Martin, B.R.; Sangalang, M.; Wu, S.; Armstrong, D.G. Outcomes of allogenic acellular matrix therapy in treatment of diabetic foot wounds: An initial experience. *Int. Wound J.* **2005**, *2*, 161–165. [CrossRef]
9. Wainwright, D.J. Use of an acellular allograft dermal matrix (AlloDerm) in the management of full-thickness burns. *Burns* **1995**, *21*, 243–248. [CrossRef]
10. Yim, H.; Cho, Y.S.; Seo, C.H.; Lee, B.C.; Ko, J.H.; Kim, D.; Hur, J.; Chun, W.; Kim, J.H. The use of AlloDerm on major burn patients: AlloDerm prevents post-burn joint contracture. *Burns* **2010**, *36*, 322–328. [CrossRef]
11. Lee, J.H.; Kim, J.-W.; Chung, K.J.; Kim, T.G.; Kim, Y.-H.; Kim, K.-J. Wound healing effects of paste type acellular dermal matrix subcutaneous injection. *Arch. Plast. Surg.* **2018**, *45*, 504–511. [CrossRef] [PubMed]
12. Marston, W.A.; Hanft, J.; Norwood, P.; Pollak, R.; Dermagraft Diabetic Foot Ulcer Study Group. The efficacy and safety of Dermagraft in improving the healing of chronic diabetic foot ulcers: Results of a prospective randomized trial. *Diabetes Care* **2003**, *26*, 1701–1705. [CrossRef] [PubMed]
13. Zelen, C.M.; Gould, L.; Serena, T.E.; Carter, M.J.; Keller, J.; Li, W.W. A prospective, randomised, controlled, multi-centre comparative effectiveness study of healing using dehydrated human amnion/chorion membrane allograft, bioengineered skin substitute or standard of care for treatment of chronic lower extremity diabetic ulcers. *Int. Wound J.* **2015**, *12*, 724–732. [PubMed]
14. Zelen, C.M.; Serena, T.E.; Gould, L.; Le, L.; Carter, M.J.; Keller, J.; Li, W.W. Treatment of chronic diabetic lower extremity ulcers with advanced therapies: A prospective, randomised, controlled, multi-centre comparative study examining clinical efficacy and cost. *Int. Wound J.* **2016**, *13*, 272–282. [CrossRef]

15. Li, R.; Guo, W.; Yang, B.; Guo, L.; Sheng, L.; Chen, G.; Li, Y.; Zou, Q.; Xie, D.; An, X.; et al. Human treated dentin matrix as a natural scaffold for complete human dentin tissue regeneration. *Biomaterials* **2011**, *32*, 4525–4538. [CrossRef]
16. Lee, M.; Jun, D.; Choi, H.; Kim, J.; Shin, D. Clinical efficacy of acellular dermal matrix paste in treating diabetic foot ulcers. *Wounds* **2020**, *32*, 50–56.
17. Kim, S.W.; Shim, H.S.; Lee, J.; Kim, Y.H. Application of paste-type acellular dermal matrix in hard-to-heal wounds. *J. Wound Care* **2021**, *30*, 414–418. [CrossRef] [PubMed]
18. Jung, J.-A.; Yoo, K.-H.; Han, S.-K.; Dhong, E.-S.; Kim, W.-K. Evaluation of the efficacy of highly hydrophilic polyurethane foam dressing in treating a diabetic foot ulcer. *Adv. Ski. Wound Care* **2016**, *29*, 546–555. [CrossRef]
19. Brigido, S.A. The use of an acellular dermal regenerative tissue matrix in the treatment of lower extremity wounds: A prospective 16-week pilot study. *Int. Wound J.* **2006**, *3*, 181–187. [CrossRef]
20. Pizzo, A.M.; Kokini, K.; Vaughn, L.C.; Waisner, B.Z.; Voytik-Harbin, S.L. Extracellular matrix (ECM) microstructural composition regulates local cell-ECM biomechanics and fundamental fibroblast behavior: A multidimensional perspective. *J. Appl. Physiol.* **2005**, *98*, 1909–1921. [CrossRef]
21. Hodde, J.; Ernst, D.; Hiles, M. An investigation of the long-term bioactivity of endogenous growth factor in OASIS Wound Matrix. *J. Wound Care* **2005**, *14*, 23–25. [CrossRef] [PubMed]
22. Hodde, J.P.; Record, R.D.; Liang, H.A.; Badylak, S.F. Vascular endothelial growth factor in porcine-derived extracellular matrix. *Endothelium* **2001**, *8*, 11–242. [CrossRef] [PubMed]
23. Brigido, S.A.; Schwartz, E.; McCarroll, R.; Hardin-Young, J. Use of an acellular flowable dermal replacement scaffold on lower extremity sinus tract wounds: A retrospective series. *Foot Ankle Spec.* **2009**, *2*, 67–72. [CrossRef] [PubMed]
24. Jeon, M.; Kim, S.Y. Application of a paste-type acellular dermal matrix for coverage of chronic ulcerative wounds. *Arch. Plast. Surg.* **2018**, *45*, 564–571. [CrossRef]
25. Nicholas, M.N.; Yeung, J. Current status and future of skin substitutes for chronic wound healing. *J. Cutan. Med. Surg.* **2017**, *21*, 23–30. [CrossRef]
26. Sen, C.K.; Gordillo, G.M.; Roy, S.; Kirsner, R.; Lambert, L.; Hunt, T.K.; Gottrup, F.; Gurtner, G.C.; Longaker, M.T. Human skin wounds: A major and snowballing threat to public health and the economy. *Wound Repair Regen.* **2009**, *17*, 763–771. [CrossRef]
27. Wu, S.C.; Driver, V.R.; Wrobel, J.S.; Armstrong, D.G. Foot ulcers in the diabetic patient, prevention and treatment. *Vasc. Health Risk Manag.* **2007**, *3*, 65–76.
28. Reyzelman, A.; Crews, R.T.; Moore, J.C.; Moore, L.; Mukker, J.S.; Offutt, S.; Tallis, A.; Turner, W.B.; Vayser, D.; Winters, C.; et al. Clinical effectiveness of an acellular dermal regenerative tissue matrix compared to standard wound management in healing diabetic foot ulcers: A prospective, randomised, multicentre study. *Int. Wound J.* **2009**, *6*, 196–208. [CrossRef]
29. Eppley, B.L. Experimental assessment of the revascularization of acellular human dermis for soft-tissue augmentation. *Plast. Reconstr. Surg.* **2001**, *107*, 757–762. [CrossRef]
30. Tognetti, L.; Pianigiani, E.; Ierardi, F.; Lorenzini, G.; Casella, D.; Liso, F.G.; De Pascalis, A.; Cinotti, E.; Rubegni, P. The use of human acellular dermal matrices in advanced wound healing and surgical procedures: State of the art. *Dermatol. Ther.* **2021**, *34*, e14987. [CrossRef]
31. Taylor, D.A.; Sampaio, L.C.; Ferdous, Z.; Gobin, A.S.; Taite, L.J. Decellularized matrices in regenerative medicine. *Acta Biomater.* **2018**, *74*, 74–89. [CrossRef] [PubMed]
32. Hahn, H.M.; Lee, D.H.; Lee, I.J. Ready-to-use micronized human acellular dermal matrix to accelerate wound healing in diabetic foot ulcers: A prospective randomized pilot study. *Adv. Ski. Wound Care* **2021**, *34*, 1–6. [CrossRef] [PubMed]

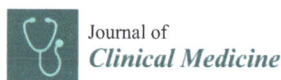

Review

The Role of the Immune System in Pediatric Burns: A Systematic Review

Tomasz Korzeniowski [1,2], Paulina Mertowska [3,*], Sebastian Mertowski [3], Martyna Podgajna [3], Ewelina Grywalska [3], Jerzy Strużyna [2,4] and Kamil Torres [1,2]

1. Chair and Department of Didactics and Medical Simulation, Medical University of Lublin, 20-093 Lublin, Poland; t.korzeniowski@gmail.com (T.K.); kamil.torres@umlub.pl (K.T.)
2. East Center of Burns Treatment and Reconstructive Surgery, 21-010 Łęczna, Poland; jerzy.struzyna@gmail.com
3. Department of Experimental Immunology, Medical University of Lublin, 20-093 Lublin, Poland; sebastian.mertowski@umlub.pl (S.M.); 50618@umlub.pl (M.P.); ewelina.grywalska@umlub.pl (E.G.)
4. Chair and Department of Plastic, Reconstructive Surgery and Burn Treatment, Medical University of Lublin, 20-093 Lublin, Poland
* Correspondence: paulina.mertowska@umlub.pl; Tel.: +48-81448-6420

Abstract: Burns are one of the most common causes of home injuries, characterized by serious damage to the skin and causing the death of affected tissues. In this review, we intended to collect information on the pathophysiological effects of burns in pediatric patients, with particular emphasis on local and systemic responses. A total of 92 articles were included in the review, and the time range of the searched articles was from 2000 to 2021. The occurrence of thermal injuries is a problem that requires special attention in pediatric patients who are still developing. Their exposure to various burns may cause disturbances in the immune response, not only in the area of tissue damage itself but also by disrupting the systemic immune response. The aspect of immunological mechanisms in burns requires further research, and in particular, it is important to focus on younger patients as the existence of subtle differences in wound healing between adults and children may significantly influence the treatment of pediatric patients.

Keywords: wound healing; burns; immune response; burn shock; immune system

1. Introduction

Burns are one of the injuries that damage not only the skin but also deeper tissues. Most often, these injuries are caused by exposure to high temperatures, overexposure to the sun or other radiation, and skin exposure to a chemical agent or electric shock (Figure 1A) [1–3]. Burns are mainly characterized by serious damage to the skin, which causes the death of the affected skin cells, which are the body's first line of defense against harmful environmental factors, injuries and infections [4,5]. The consequences of a high temperature on human skin (depending on the temperature and duration of exposure) may lead not only to local but also systemic damage [6–10]. According to the information presented by the World Health Organization (WHO) and the Center for Disease Prevention and Control (CDC), burns are one of the most common causes of home injuries, and children under 19 are particularly vulnerable [11,12]. As shown in the literature, burns are one of the causes of the loss of Disability Adjusted Life Years (DALYs), mainly in middle- and low-income countries (with a DALY of 96 per 100,000) [13,14]. However, burns are not only a significant cause of increased morbidity and disability among children but also one of the major causes of death in this group of patients. According to WHO data, nearly 180,000 people die from burns each year [11,15]. Although child mortality rates have declined in recent years, this trend only applies to highly developed countries, e.g., in the United States, the death rate of children due to burns fell from 0.71 per 100,000 in 2004 to 0.39 per 100,000 in 2018 [16,17]. Still, the percentage of children dying from burns in low-

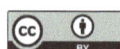

and middle-income countries is almost 11 times higher than in highly developed countries and amounts to 4.3 deaths per 100,000 [18,19]. Moreover, the available literature data also show that the highest risk group for burns is children aged 0–4 years, among whom the mortality rate of 0.71 per 100,000 deaths was recorded in the United States in 2018. This is 1.45× higher than the group of children aged 5–9 and 2.84× higher than that of children aged 10–14 and also 5.46× higher than of adolescents aged 15–19 (Figure 1B). Undoubtedly, such a discrepancy results from stages of child development in individual age groups and their self-awareness, as children up to the age of 4 begin to move independently on their own and are extremely curious about the world [16,20]. Additionally, medical reports analyzed by the WHO show that male patients are hospitalized much more often as a result of burns than females. These tendencies are confirmed by the collected data, which show that in each age group, men are more likely to get burns, accounting for about 57% of eruptions registered cases (Figure 1C) [16,21]. Retrospective studies conducted by the American Academy of Pediatrics showed that the development of the COVID-19 pandemic also contributed to the increase in the number of burns among children under the age of 19. The presented data show that in 2020, there was a rise in pediatric patients with burns by 48.6% compared to the year 2019 (Figure 1D). The highest increase was observed in the age group 10–14 (by 103.85% compared to 2019) and in the groups of 5–9 years (an increase of 55.88%) and 1–4 years (an increase by 56.11%) (Figure 1D). As researchers point out, this is undoubtedly due to the prolonged stay of children at home as a result of the introduction of remote learning [22].

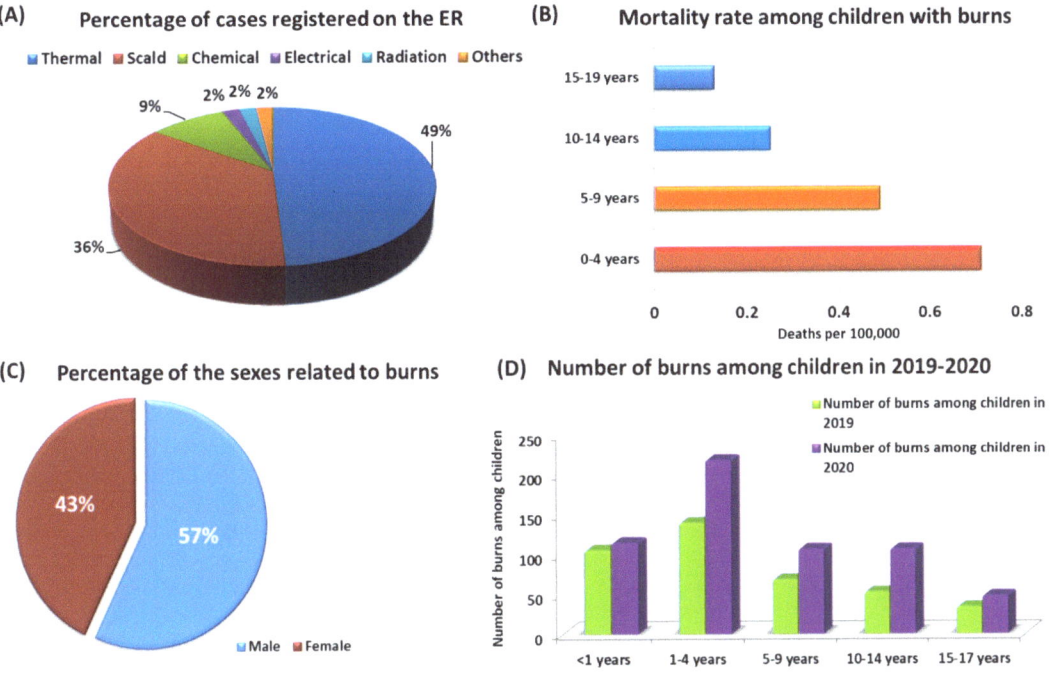

Figure 1. Statistics of burns among children: (A) percentage of burns recorded in the ER, including the cause of the injury; (B) child mortality rate as a result of burns by age category; (C) percentage of burns by patient's sex; (D) number of burns among children in 2019–2020, taking into account age categories based on [16,18,22].

Children are a special group of patients in whom burns are associated with much greater and more serious consequences than in the case of adults. First, these differences are due to the structure of the skin itself, which is much thinner in children than in adults. This means that both the time and energy required to cause a burn in children is shorter than in adults, resulting in injuries that occur much faster and are also deeper than in adults. It also leads to several local or systemic changes in such patients who are exposed to wound infections, prolonged healing, hypothermia, development of severe inflammatory reactions, hypermetabolic syndrome, and immunosuppression [23–25]. Damage to the skin as a result of burns leads to dysregulation, the loss of the protective barrier, but also neurosensory and metabolic functions (disturbances in water homeostasis and thermoregulation), as well as immunological functions are impaired. The immune system plays an extremely important role in the body's response to burns, determining the prognosis and recovery time for many patients, especially pediatric ones. Tissue damage during a burn causes a strong inflammatory reaction, leading to impaired immune function. Extensive inflammation developing in children up to 19 years of age causes the release of inflammatory mediators and markers, the accumulation of which may cause systemic inflammatory response syndrome (SIRS), which in turn leads to dysregulation of the immune homeostasis of the human body but also to the development of multiple organ dysfunction syndrome (MODS) [26–28]. Burn-induced changes affect the functioning of many immunological cells and the compounds they secrete (mainly cytokines), which impair the innate and acquired mechanisms of the patient's immune system [29]. SIRS developing in the patient's body contributes to the increase in immunosuppression, which makes the body more susceptible to bacterial infections and the development of sepsis [30]. Additionally, the hyperinflammatory reaction observed in the course of sepsis leads to the formation of the state of "immunoparalysis" in the body, which is particularly dangerous in pediatric patients [31]. The immunoparalysis syndrome can affect both innate and adaptive mechanisms of immune responses, in which reduced HLA-DR expression is observed in monocytes, as well as the reduced ability to produce cytokines by leukocytes, the presence of lymphopenia, and the increased expression of inhibitory immune checkpoints on the cell surface such as PD-1 [32–35].

The detailed role of the immune system and the specific immune cells and its importance in the evolution of tissue changes in burns is an extremely important research topic aimed at a better understanding of the mechanisms influencing the healing of injuries and restoring the immune balance. The purpose of this review is to gather information on the pathophysiological effects of burns in pediatric patients, with particular emphasis on local and systemic responses. In addition, we would like to present the important role of the immune system in the course of burns and the healing process of this type of injury, which, as a result of dysregulation of the mechanisms of innate and acquired responses, leads to immunosuppression that threatens life and health of children.

2. Materials and Methods

Search Strategy, Study Selection, and Data Extraction

The literature analysis was carried out on the PubMed database where the search for available articles was performed based on the following keywords: "Burns in children", "Pediatric burns", "Paediatric burns", "Immunity", "Immune response", "Immune system". The time range of the searched articles was established for the years 2000 to 2021, and filters related to the type of articles (clinical trials, review, systematic review, book) were used. Repetitions were rejected from the found articles. The suitability for the inclusion of each work into the publication was thoroughly assessed. Eventually, 88 articles were included in the review.

3. Assessment of the Effects of Burns in Pediatric Patients

Burns are an extremely dynamic type of damage to the body, the scale of which in the initial stages after contact with the agent is difficult to estimate due to the problems with assessing the depth and extent of the resulting wounds on the patient's body [36]. The speed of assessing the severity of such an injury (burn size, percentage of burnt the body surface, fluid resuscitation) influences the selection of the appropriate clinical procedure and its subsequent consequences (development of inflammation, hypermetabolic syndrome, tissue infections or risk of death), especially in the case of pediatric patients [37].

The size of burns in children will be different in relation to adults due to changes in the percentage of the patient's body surface area resulting from their individual development. There are several methods of counting the extent of burns, expressed as a percentage of the total body surface area [19,38]. Typically, adolescents (over 14 years of age) and adults use the "rule of nine", with each upper limb accounting for 9% and each lower limb accounting for 18% of the total body surface area. Additionally, the head accounts for 9%, the torso for 18%, and the perineum for 1% of the total body surface [39,40].

Contrary to the rule of nines, the Lund and Browder chart is used very often to assess the extent of burns in pediatric patients, which considers the age of the burned person [41]. It characterizes particular regions of the pediatric patient's body in detail, where the percentage of burns to the head decreases and the percentage of burns to the legs increases with the age of a child, which makes it a much more effective tool for assessing the extent of burns in such patients [42].

3.1. Pathophysiological Effects of Burns in Pediatric Patients

The consequences of burns lead to the loss of basic functions of the skin, which is thinner in children than in adults. Additionally, children have an increased metabolism, increased heat loss (conditioned by lower body fat content) and are exposed to increased water loss due to evaporation [43]. The effects of burns in pediatric patients are undoubtedly more dangerous and burdened with a higher risk of complications than in adults. Younger children are at risk of developing hypothermia and increased evaporation loss due to a greater surface area to weight ratio [44]. There is also an increased risk of damage or obstruction of the airways (due to the smaller opening of the airways), possible laryngeal edema, sepsis, hypervolemia or dysfunction of internal organs (heart or kidneys) [45–47]. The inflammatory reaction following burns in pediatric patients is also usually stronger than in adults, which is also associated with increased susceptibility to the development of a hypermetabolic state [48]. Due to the fact that children are still in the growth period, the management of wounds or scarring caused by burns is an additional compilation, as the applied treatments must allow the skin to grow and maintain its elasticity in order to adapt to each stage of the patient's development [24].

All pathophysiological effects and consequences of burns occurring in pediatric patients can be divided into local and systemic reactions [10,49].

3.1.1. Local Response to Burns in Pediatric Patients

Thermal injuries that cause burns occur in the human body in two characteristic stages. First, coagulation-type necrosis develops in the epidermis and tissues. This is an acute type of necrosis that causes degeneration of protein fibers, turning albumin into an opaque, compact structure. Structural proteins are also denatured, which results in the inhibition of proteolytic activity [50]. The next step is cell lysis damage that occurs as a result of the progression of ischemic skin damage (24–48 h), caused by the development of vascular thrombosis [51,52]. Within the cells of the immune system, platelets and leukocytes adhere to the surface of the vascular endothelium, while in the complement system, cytotoxic T lymphocytes (Tc) are activated, and the burn tissue itself develops into a site open to various types of infections [53]. There are also several local lesions within the skin as a result of burns. Three distinctive regions are formed: the coagulation (necrosis) zone, the stagnant (ischemic) zone, and the outermost hyperthermic (inflammatory) zone [54]. In the first zone, structural proteins coagulate, causing irreversible tissue damage. In the second one, tissue perfusion decreases, but the cells present in this area are still alive, and the application of a treatment that increases tissue perfusion may save them. Within the third zone, tissue perfusion is increased, and the blood vessels develop characteristic dilation due to the development of inflammation surrounding the burn. Clinical data show that tissues in this area require 7–10 days to regenerate, which may be prolonged when infection occurs [55,56].

3.1.2. Systemic Response to Burns in Pediatric Patients

The systemic response to burns affects almost all internal organs of the patient's body (e.g., heart, kidney, liver). In severe burns, cytokines and other inflammatory mediators are released in excess in both burn and non-burn areas. These mediators cause narrowing and dilation of blood vessels, an increase in capillary permeability, and the development of edema both at the burn site and in distant organs. Pathological changes also occur in the metabolic, cardiovascular, renal, gastrointestinal and coagulation systems (Figure 2) [47,57,58].

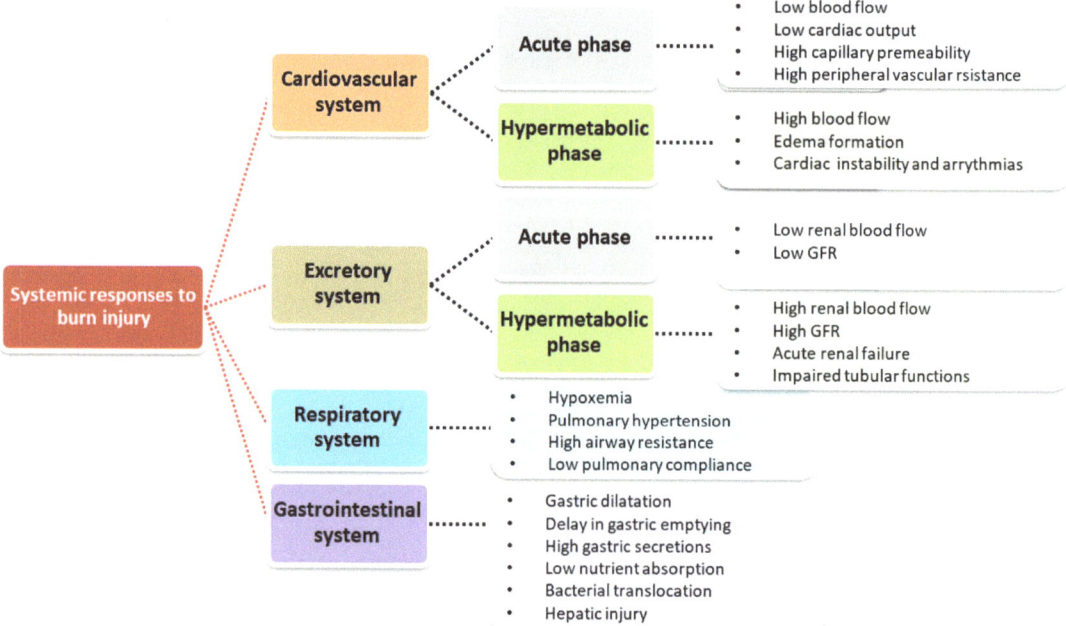

Figure 2. Systemic response to burn injury based on [47].

The extensive inflammatory reaction of the body to burns can alter the immune response. Here, we can observe the formation of a pro-inflammatory phase that results in the development of SIRS, as well as an anti-inflammatory phase, known as the compensatory anti-inflammatory response syndrome (CARS). Only the balance of these two phases will guarantee therapeutic success. Otherwise, developing SIRS or CARS responses will lead to the development of MODS, infection, sepsis, and even death of the patient (Figure 3).

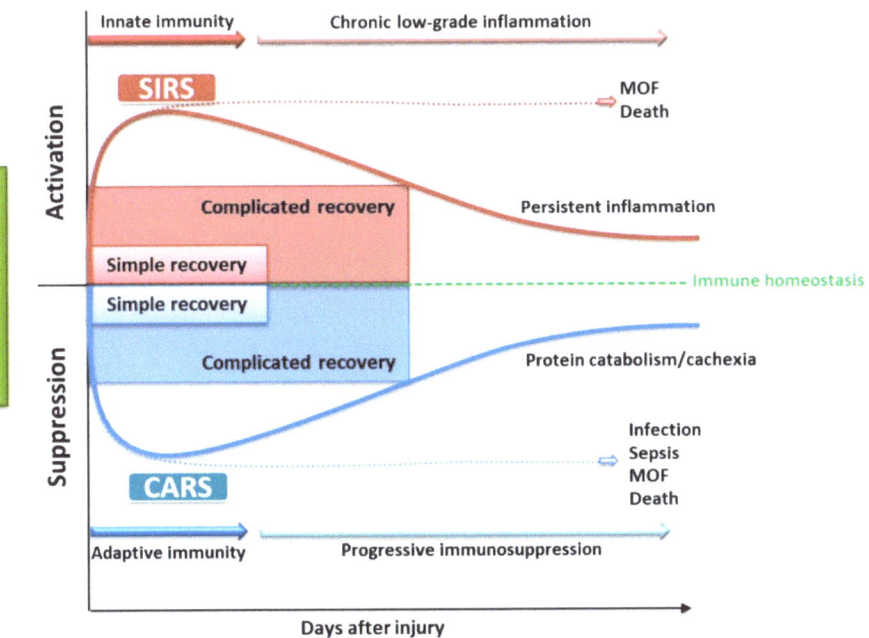

Figure 3. Importance of maintaining immune homeostasis in burns based on [59,60].

3.1.3. Burn Shock

When the area of burn of the body exceeds 30%, the body releases kinins from the burn area into the bloodstream (histamine, bradykinin, serotonin) and inflammatory mediators, e.g., cytokines and thromboxanes, prostacyclins, prostaglandins, or leukotrienes, which, when reaching high levels, cause a systemic response [61]. This leads to damage to the endothelium and, consequently, to the displacement of fluids between individual fluid spaces. Plasma finds its way into both tissues damaged by burns and healthy ones. As a result of these processes, the amount of fluid in the vascular bed decreases rapidly, and therefore, burn shock occurs. The burn shock period can be examined in three periods: early, intermediate, and late [62,63].

The first of these, also known as the seepage period, covers the first 36–72 h after the onset of the injury. Then, blood vessels dilate at the burn site, which is accompanied by the release of systemic inflammatory mediators such as histamine, TNF-α, IL-1, IL-6, GM-CSF, INF-γ, or prostaglandins, which are secreted not only from the places of injury themselves but also from healthy tissues adjacent to the burn [64]. The shock generated after the burn is hypovolemic and directly proportional to the extent and severity of the burn. As shown in the literature, in adults, burns of 20% of the body surface area lead to an increased risk of developing hypervolemic shock. In pediatric patients, especially in children under 12, the percentage of body surface burns that correlate with the increased possibility of developing hypervolemic shock is reduced and amounts to 10% [65,66]. Hypovolemia due to circulatory fluid loss caused by edema is observed within the first 2 days and leads to the development of hemodynamic failure due to reduced blood volume [67]. The most common clinical symptoms that indicate the development of hypervolemic shock are pale, moist, and cool skin; tachycardia and hypotension; rapid and shallow breathing; and reduction in urine volume [67,68].

The next period is the intermediate period, also known as the intoxication period, which covers the span of 2 to 4 weeks after the burn occurs [69]. During this time, edema formation ceases, and denatured proteins released from cells enter the circulation, creating a case of intoxication in the body [63]. Approximately 7 days after the injury, the patient's hemodynamic situation is reversed, accompanied by abnormally high cardiac output and vasodilation [70]. One of the characteristic symptoms of this stage is the appearance of polyuria [71].

The last period of burn shock is the infectious period, in which acute or chronic infections may occur [69]. Both the cellular and humoral immune responses are suppressed at this stage depending on the body surface area that has been damaged by the burn. This leads to the development of lymphopenia, which affects the processes of chemotaxis and phagocytosis [72,73]. Depending on the degree of burn, the activation of T lymphocytes is also weakened, which makes the human body more predisposed/vulnerable to bacterial, viral, or fungal infections [74]. The profiles of cytokines produced by immune cells are also changing, including IL-2, IL-1, IL-6, and IL-8, the concentration of which decreases significantly in the first weeks after the onset of injury, as shown by literature data [63,75,76]. Additionally, increased cell catabolism and the occurrence of capillary leakage reduce the circulating levels of immunoglobulins (IgG, IgA, and IgM) in the peripheral blood [77,78]. Studies by Sobouti et al. show that the decrease in serum immunoglobulin levels is independent of the size of the burn in children. However, they showed that more severe burns in patients were associated with greater reductions in serum levels of IgA, IgM, IgG, and their subclasses [77].

4. The Role of the Immune System in Burns

In burn injuries, the wound healing response is characterized by three stages: inflammation, cell proliferation, and subsequent remodeling. In the first stage, innate immunity is involved, which is triggered by the release of factors such as histamine or cytokines, which cause the expansion of blood vessels, allowing the first line of defense cells such as neutrophils, monocytes, or macrophages to reach the site of damage [79]. The initiated inflammatory process plays an important role in healing burn wounds, as cells such as neutrophils, monocytes, and macrophages can stimulate the activity of fibroblasts and keratinocytes in the proliferation and remodeling phase [79]. Many cells of the immune system are involved in the process of healing wounds resulting from burns, the basic functions of which are presented in Figure 4. All disorders of the immune response at the stage of the healing process of burn wounds may lead to immunosuppression and increased predisposition of patients to various types of infections, which will significantly affect the recovery time [58]. That is why it is so important to establish the mechanisms and functioning of the immune system in patients with burns.

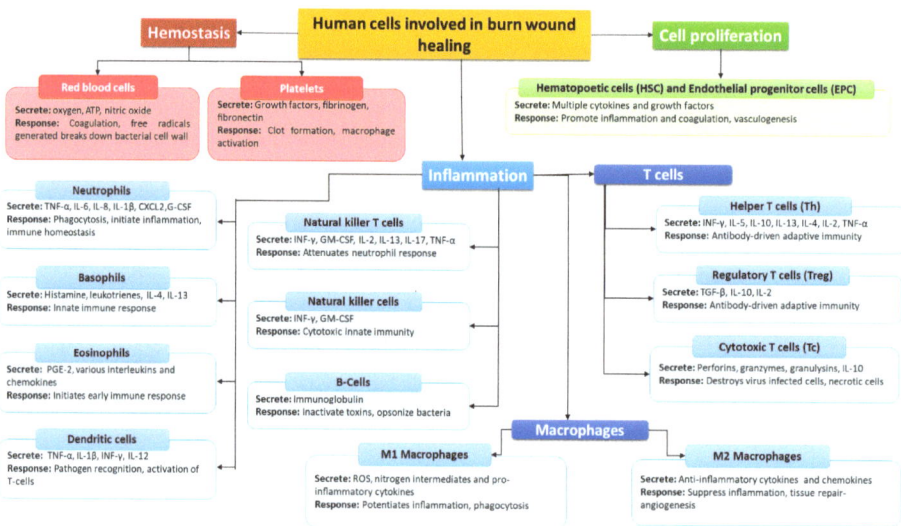

Figure 4. Human cells involved in burn wound healing based on [79–82].

4.1. Importance of the Innate Response (Neutrophils, Monocytes, Macrophages, NK Cells)

One of the most important elements of innate immunity in the event of burns is the triggering of a pro-inflammatory cascade caused by thermal trauma. Starting this process may also have significant consequences leading to complications; therefore, determining the participation of individual cells in the process is important [58]. Literature data focusing on the burn area indicate that monocytes, which can transform into macrophages, are important cells involved in the above-mentioned processes. Monocytes and macrophages are involved in immune processes related to phagocytosis (capture and absorption of molecules), including foreign antigens and harmful microorganisms, which include bacteria, viruses and fungi. Macrophages participate in transport of iron to the body tissues, support the production of antibodies and blood vessel formation. Monocytes, although they constitute only a small percentage of all leukocytes, are therefore extremely important for the body [48]. As a result of recognition of molecular patterns, these cells are activated, which in turn leads to the production of chemokines and cytokines [57]. The main mediators secreted by activated monocytes include TNF-α, IL-6 and IL-1β, and IL-10 [57].

The secretion of such compounds influences the mechanism of regulation of the immune and acute phase of response to trauma. In the case of TNF-α, it is involved in the development of a shock-like state associated with thermal damage and sepsis, while IL-1 and IL-6, through their actions, will lead to the activation of granulocytes and the proliferation of T and B lymphocytes [58]. In addition to the above-mentioned mechanisms, activated monocytes, through antigen presentation and expression of, e.g., HLA-DR molecules, can bind to lymphocytes, as a result of which T cells can become activated. In addition, it is indicated that the percentage of monocytes with HLA-DR on their surface is lower in burn patients compared to the control group and is lowest in burn patients who developed sepsis [57]. Monocytes and their subsets (classical subsets of approximately 85 to 95% and intermediate and non-classical subsets of approximately 5 and 9% of all monocytes) play an extremely important role in wound healing. The most important of them seems to be the intermediate subpopulation, which shows high expression of surface markers, such as endothelial growth factors I and II and CXCR4 (C-X-C Motif Chemokine Receptor 4). In addition, as indicated in the literature, this subset after trauma can produce large amounts of proinflammatory cytokines (such as tumor necrosis factor and IL-12), increased levels of which have been detected in severe infections. However, despite extensive research, the role of individual monocyte subsets in burn healing remains unclear [83]. In the case of burns, macrophages play an equally important role as other cells of the immune system and a major role in removing dead cells through phagocytosis. The action of these contributes to stimulating inflammation, but they also secrete compounds that stimulate the healing process of injury, such as fibroblast growth factor, vascular endothelial growth factor, or platelet-derived growth factor [84]. The secretion of the abovementioned factors supports the angiogenesis process. In addition, in the process of wound formation at the stage of proliferation, macrophages produce proteases and stimulate the migration of endothelial cells through the fibroblast growth factor and the production of TGF-β. In addition to supporting the human body in the process of regenerating a burn injury, macrophages also play an important role in defense against pathogens. The performance of so many functions by macrophages is possible thanks to their adaptive function depending on the environment. We can distinguish two types of macrophages: M1 and M2. The first is activated in the classical way; they are used to fight pathogens and are called inflammatory macrophages due to the stimulation of inflammation. In contrast, M2 macrophages are activated by alternative routes depending on the received stimuli from the environment. Due to this ability, they can perform various functions related to the repair of damaged tissues, and they can secrete compounds that reduce inflammation. As a result of thermal damage in wound healing, the phenotype of M1 cells may change to M2 [48,83].

Neutrophils are the next cells involved in the innate immune response. These cells use, e.g., phagolysosomes, free radicals release, or antimicrobial proteases in order to fight pathogens [48]. Neutrophils are also the next cells that migrate the fastest to the burn injury site. However, they show reduced chemotaxis, phagocytosis, and decreased bactericidal capacity, which leads to, despite their relatively large number in burn wounds, impairment of their effector function [48,57]. Reduced neutrophil chemotaxis after a burn can be induced by ceramide-mediated chemotaxis inhibition [84]. As cells of innate immunity, neutrophils can quickly react directly to pathogens by following chemoattractants such as interleukins, chemokines, or bacterial antigens that determine the path that neutrophils are to follow. Weakened neutrophil migration can be supported using antibiotics [57]. Neutrophils, in addition to the function of eliminating pathogens, participate in the process of tissue cleansing. Like monocytes, these cells secrete pro-inflammatory cytokines TNF-α, IL-1β, and IL-6, which indicate the damaged area to other cells, which in turn contributes to the migration of other cells of the immune system to the burned area [48].

Other cells involved in the host's defense during thermal damage are NK cells (natural killers). These cells are characterized by high cytolytic activity from releasing cytotoxic granules that attach, for example, to infected cells and induce programmed cell death [79]. Rapid response to pathogens (mainly viral) and to abnormal self and infected cells is based on the ability of these cells to kill without recognition of the histocompatibility complex [57]. This type of cell is especially important in burn patients as it enables a rapid response to viral infections that can significantly increase the mortality rate of these patients [57]. NK cells are activated by type I interferon (IFN) and type III interferons. Upon activation, these cells induce the synthesis of type II interferons, IFN-γ and TNF-α [79]. Unfortunately, as a result of thermal damage, despite the unchanged percentage of NK cells, their functioning in the body may be impaired. In the case of pediatric patients, there are no studies available in the literature addressing this aspect, and the limitation of NK cell function has currently only been detected in adult patients. Scientific research shows that a decrease in NK cell activity is observed in burn patients with more than 20% of the total body surface area (TBSA) compared to those with a smaller burn area [57]. The probable mechanism of action of these cells presented in scientific studies is related to the level of IL-2. The lower amount of this interleukin correlates with the lower activity of NK cells. It is also indicated that this correlation may be typical for burn injuries as this type of phenomenon is not detected in people with injuries other than burns [57,58].

4.2. Importance of the Acquired Response

Another type of host reaction to burns is the involvement of cells responsible for the acquired immunity, such as lymphocytes. As in the case of innate immune cells, several changes can occur as a result of burns in lymphocytes. One such process may be lymphocyte suppression [57]. In the course of burns, helper T lymphocytes (Th lymphocytes), regulatory T lymphocytes (Treg), and gamma-delta T lymphocytes ($\gamma\delta$) are important subpopulations [57]. According to research data, the skin and epithelial tissues are dominated by a subpopulation of $\gamma\delta$ T lymphocytes that express $\gamma\delta$ T lymphocyte receptors ($\gamma\delta$ TCR) [79]. These cells are also likely to be an important source of chemokines as well as pro-inflammatory cytokines. Additionally, these cells recruit marrow cells to the burn wound to regulate local inflammation [57,79]. T helper lymphocytes can be divided, among others, into subtypes Th1 and Th2. Each type of cell is responsible for a different function: Th1 cells are usually assigned a pro-inflammatory role, while Th2 cells are assigned an anti-inflammatory function. The formation of the Th1 subpopulation is stimulated by IL-12, while the differentiation into Th2 cells is induced by IL-4. As a result of burn damage, the dominant subpopulation in the damaged area is the Th2 type [57]. Another subtype is Treg cells, which are antagonized by Th17 cells. Tregs are regulating cells, including the process of T lymphocyte proliferation, as a result of which, they play an important role in inducing tolerance to transplanted tissue and reducing the inflammatory response. Their action also influences the immune response after burn injuries. According to the literature, these cells are characterized by increased function and occurrence in the lymph nodes after burns. In animal models, it was also observed that the lack of Treg lymphocytes increased the response induced by Th1 lymphocytes [57]. Th17 lymphocytes are a subpopulation of T cells with an antagonistic effect on Treg cells. They act in the recruitment and activation of neutrophils and are responsible for the secretion of IL-17 and IL-22, thus demonstrating a strong pro-inflammatory effect. In children, compared to adults, the level of IL-17 in the early stages after a burn is higher. This may indicate a different IL-17 expression profile compared to adults. This allows for a hypothesis about the existence of differences in the immune system functioning in pediatric patients after burns compared to adult patients; however, this conclusion requires deeper analysis and confirmation in other studies [57].

There is very little information in the literature on the role of B lymphocytes in burns. It is important to mention their lower activity, accompanied by a lower concentration of immunoglobulins in the serum of patients after thermal injuries [57].

Another mechanism that may influence the immune response is co-inhibitory molecules whose task is to regulate the immune response and in particular to suppress this response. Such molecules include the programmed death 1 (PD-1) molecule with its ligands and the CTLA-4 molecule.

The PD-1 molecule is a molecule found on the cell surface. The presence of PD-1 is mainly observed on T lymphocytes and acts as a checkpoint for them as it indicates their condition and state of exhaustion [85]. When the PD-1 receptor binds to its ligands (PD-L1 or PD-L2) on antigen-presenting cells, the pro-inflammatory response is inhibited and results in the process of lymphocyte apoptosis on which this molecule was expressed [57,86]. In the case of burns, an increased expression of the PD-1 molecule has been shown, which may reduce the number of T lymphocytes.

On the other hand, the CTLA-4 molecule is most frequently expressed on T lymphocytes and has an influence on the suppression of the immune response. This molecule belongs to the immunoglobulin subfamily CD28, and its ligands are the receptors CD80 and CD86 on the surface of antigen-presenting cells [87]. Additionally, the CTLA-4 receptor competes with the CD28 molecule to associate with its ligands. As a result of this mechanism and depending on the binding of ligands to this molecule or to its antagonist receptor, the stimulation or inhibition of the immune response of T-lymphocytes may occur. Therefore, CTLA-4 is considered an important factor that allows the maintenance of T-cell homeostasis and their autotolerance to it [87]. As in the case of PD-1 and in relation to the CTLA-4 molecule, it can be viewed as the so-called immune checkpoint. In the case of this receptor, in studies on cancer patients and in patients with viral infections, an improvement in the immune response was achieved after treatment aimed at blocking this molecule. This could indicate that this molecule could also be a potential therapeutic target in the event of burns [57,87].

5. Conclusions

The occurrence of thermal injuries is a problem that requires special attention in the case of pediatric patients whose bodies are still developing. Exposing young people to burns (depending on the degree of damage) may cause disturbances in the immune response, not only in the area of tissue damage itself but also in the systemic immune response. Developing severe inflammation caused by thermal trauma may affect the entire body, disrupting the immune homeostasis and affecting the entire process of wound healing and convalescence, as well as the occurrence of severe complications. Therefore, the treatment of burns is complex and requires a holistic approach to the treated patient. Apart from the local treatment of lesions of damaged skin, nutritional and pharmacological support of the whole human body seems to be equally important, as burn patients may show a weaker immune response to infections. To summarize, the aspect of immunological mechanisms in burns requires further research, and in particular, it is important to focus on younger patients. Although the mechanisms of wound healing and responses to burns are similar in adults and children, the existence of subtle differences may significantly influence the treatment of pediatric patients.

Author Contributions: Conceptualization, T.K., E.G. and K.T.; methodology, T.K., P.M., S.M., M.P., E.G. and K.T.; software, T.K., P.M., S.M., M.P., E.G. and K.T.; validation, T.K., P.M., S.M., M.P., E.G. and K.T.; formal analysis, T.K., P.M., S.M., M.P., E.G. and K.T.; investigation, T.K., P.M., S.M., M.P., E.G. and K.T.; resources, P.M. and S.M.; data curation, T.K., P.M., S.M., M.P., E.G. and K.T.; writing—original draft preparation, T.K., P.M., S.M. and M.P.; writing—review and editing, E.G., J.S. and K.T.; visualization, P.M. and S.M.; supervision, E.G., J.S. and K.T.; project administration, T.K., P.M., S.M., M.P., E.G. and K.T.; funding acquisition, K.T. All authors have read and agreed to the published version of the manuscript.

Funding: This research was funded by the Medical University of Lublin, grants no. DS495 and no. GI10.

Institutional Review Board Statement: Not applicable.

Informed Consent Statement: Not applicable.

Data Availability Statement: Not applicable.

Conflicts of Interest: The authors declare no conflict of interest.

References

1. National Institute of General Medical Sciences. Burns. Available online: https://www.nigms.nih.gov/education/fact-sheets/Pages/burns.aspx (accessed on 21 February 2022).
2. Practical Handbook for Burns Injury Management (Draft).Pdf. Available online: https://dghs.gov.in/WriteReadData/userfiles/file/Comp-2/Practical%20handbook%20for%20burns%20injury%20management%20(draft).pdf (accessed on 13 March 2022).
3. Ja, G.-E.; Vb, A.-A.; Eh, O.-V.; García-Manzano, R.; Barker Antonio, A.; Aron, J.; García-Espinoza, J. Burns: Definition, Classification, Pathophysiology and Initial Approach. *Int. J. Gen. Med.* **2020**, *5*, 2327–5146. [CrossRef]
4. Skin Microbes and the Immune Response. Available online: https://www.nih.gov/news-events/nih-research-matters/skin-microbes-immune-response (accessed on 21 February 2022).
5. Padbury, J.F. Skin—The first line of defense. *J. Pediatr.* **2008**, *152*, A2. [CrossRef]
6. Chen, C.-P.; Hwang, R.-L.; Chang, S.-Y.; Lu, Y.-T. Effects of temperature steps on human skin physiology and thermal sensation response. *Build. Environ.* **2011**, *46*, 2387–2397. [CrossRef]
7. Denda, M.; Sokabe, T.; Fukumi-Tominaga, T.; Tominaga, M. Effects of Skin Surface Temperature on Epidermal Permeability Barrier Homeostasis. *J. Investig. Dermatol.* **2007**, *127*, 654–659. [CrossRef]
8. Connie, J.; Mattera, M.S. RN, EMT-P NCH Paramedic Program. Burns/Thermal Trauma. Available online: http://www.nwcemss.org/assets/1/continuing_education_materials/BURNS_thermal_S19.pdf (accessed on 13 March 2022).
9. Lévesque, B.; Lavoie, M.; Joly, J. Residential water heater temperature: 49 or 60 degrees Celsius? *Can. J. Infect. Dis.* **2004**, *15*, 11–12. [CrossRef]
10. Hettiaratchy, S.; Dziewulski, P. ABC of burns: Pathophysiology and types of burns. *BMJ* **2004**, *328*, 1427–1429. [CrossRef]
11. World Health Organization. Media Centre, Fact Sheet, Burns. January 2018. Available online: https://www.who.int/news-room/fact-sheets/detail/burns (accessed on 21 February 2022).
12. CDC Child Injury Prevention. Available online: https://www.cdc.gov/injury/features/child-injury/index.html (accessed on 21 February 2022).
13. Lyons, R.; Turner, S.; Walters, A.; Kisser, R.; Rogmans, W.; Lyons, J.; Akbari, A.; Valkenberg, H.; Bejko, D.; Bauer, R.; et al. *Disability Adjusted Life Year (DALY) Estimates for Injury Utilising the European Injury Data Base (IDB)*; LIH: Luxwembourg, 2017.
14. Spronk, I.; Edgar, D.W.; Van Baar, M.E.; Wood, F.M.; Van Loey, N.E.E.; Middelkoop, E.; Renneberg, B.; Öster, C.; Orwelius, L.; Moi, A.L.; et al. Improved and standardized method for assessing years lived with disability after burns and its application to estimate the non-fatal burden of disease of burn injuries in Australia, New Zealand and the Netherlands. *BMC Public Health* **2020**, *20*, 1–15. [CrossRef]
15. Alipour, J.; Mehdipour, Y.; Karimi, A. Epidemiology and outcome analysis of 3030 burn patients with an ICD-10 approach. *Ann. Burn. Fire Disasters* **2020**, *33*, 3–13.
16. Fire and Burn Injuries Among Children in 2018 (2020 Update). Available online: https://www.safekids.org/fast-fact/fire-and-burn-injuries-among-children-2018-2020-update (accessed on 21 February 2022).
17. World Health Organization Violence. *Injuries and Disability: Biennial Report 2010–2011*; World Health Organization: Geneva, Switzerland, 2012; ISBN 978-92-4-150413-3.
18. Peden, M.; Oyegbite, K.; Ozanne-Smith, J.; Hyder, A.A.; Branche, C.; Rahman, A.; Rivara, F.; Bartolomeos, K. *World Report on Child Injury Prevention*; WHO: Geneva, Switzerland, 2008; Chapter 2.
19. Trauma Service: Burns. Available online: https://www.rch.org.au/trauma-service/manual/Burns/ (accessed on 21 February 2022).
20. Beaulieu, E.; Zheng, A.; Rajabali, F.; MacDougall, F.; Pike, I. The Economics of Burn Injuries Among Children Aged 0 to 4 Years in British Columbia. *J. Burn Care Res.* **2020**, *42*, 499–504. [CrossRef]

21. Blom, L.; Klingberg, A.; Laflamme, L.; Wallis, L.; Hasselberg, M. Gender differences in burns: A study from emergency centres in the Western Cape, South Africa. *Burns* **2016**, *42*, 1600–1608. [CrossRef]
22. Accidental Burns Increased for Children at Home During Pandemic. Available online: http://www.aap.org/en/news-room/news-releases/aap/2021/accidental-burns-increased-for-children-at-home-during-pandemic/ (accessed on 21 February 2022).
23. Benson, A.; Dickson, W.; Boyce, D. Burns. *BMJ* **2006**, *332*, 649–652. [CrossRef]
24. Mathias, E.; Murthy, M.S. Pediatric Thermal Burns and Treatment: A Review of Progress and Future Prospects. *Medicines* **2017**, *4*, 91. [CrossRef]
25. Chipp, E.; Charles, L.; Thomas, C.; Whiting, K.; Moiemen, N.; Wilson, Y. A prospective study of time to healing and hypertrophic scarring in paediatric burns: Every day counts. *Burn. Trauma* **2017**, *5*, 3. [CrossRef]
26. Farina, J.A.; Rosique, M.J.; Rosique, R.G. Curbing Inflammation in Burn Patients. *Int. J. Inflamm.* **2013**, *2013*, 1–9. [CrossRef]
27. Greenhalgh, D.G. Sepsis in the burn patient: A different problem than sepsis in the general population. *Burn. Trauma* **2017**, *5*, 23. [CrossRef]
28. Feng, J.-Y.; Chien, J.-Y.; Kao, K.-C.; Tsai, C.-L.; Hung, F.M.; Lin, F.-M.; Hu, H.-C.; Huang, K.-L.; Yu, C.-J.; Yang, K.-Y. Predictors of Early Onset Multiple Organ Dysfunction in Major Burn Patients with Ventilator Support: Experience from A Mass Casualty Explosion. *Sci. Rep.* **2018**, *8*, 10939. [CrossRef]
29. Moins-Teisserenc, H.; Cordeiro, D.J.; Audigier, V.; Ressaire, Q.; Benyamina, M.; Lambert, J.; Maki, G.; Homyrda, L.; Toubert, A.; Legrand, M. Severe Altered Immune Status After Burn Injury Is Associated with Bacterial Infection and Septic Shock. *Front. Immunol.* **2021**, *12*. [CrossRef]
30. Zhang, P.; Zou, B.; Liou, Y.-C.; Huang, C. The pathogenesis and diagnosis of sepsis post burn injury. *Burn. Trauma* **2021**, *9*, tkaa047. [CrossRef]
31. Hall, M.W.; Greathouse, K.C.; Thakkar, R.K.; Sribnick, E.A.; Muszynski, J.A. Immunoparalysis in Pediatric Critical Care. *Pediatr. Clin. N. Am.* **2017**, *64*, 1089–1102. [CrossRef]
32. Winkler, M.S.; Rissiek, A.; Priefler, M.; Schwedhelm, E.; Robbe, L.; Bauer, A.; Zahrte, C.; Zoellner, C.; Kluge, S.; Nierhaus, A. Human leucocyte antigen (HLA-DR) gene expression is reduced in sepsis and correlates with impaired TNFα response: A diagnostic tool for immunosuppression? *PLoS ONE* **2017**, *12*, e0182427. [CrossRef]
33. Nakamori, Y.; Park, E.J.; Shimaoka, M. Immune Deregulation in Sepsis and Septic Shock: Reversing Immune Paralysis by Targeting PD-1/PD-L1 Pathway. *Front. Immunol.* **2021**, *11*, 624279. [CrossRef]
34. Berlot, G.; Passero, S. *Immunoparalysis in Septic Shock Patients*; IntechOpen: London, UK, 2019; ISBN 978-1-83880-394-0.
35. Jensen, I.J.; Sjaastad, F.V.; Griffith, T.S.; Badovinac, V.P. Sepsis-Induced T Cell Immunoparalysis: The Ins and Outs of Impaired T Cell Immunity. *J. Immunol.* **2018**, *200*, 1543–1553. [CrossRef]
36. Burn Evaluation: MedlinePlus Medical Test. Available online: https://medlineplus.gov/lab-tests/burn-evaluation/ (accessed on 21 February 2022).
37. Schaefer, T.J.; Szymanski, K.D. *Burn Evaluation and Management*; StatPearls Publishing: Treasure Island, FL, USA, 2022.
38. Suman, A.; Owen, J. Update on the management of burns in paediatrics. *BJA Educ.* **2020**, *20*, 103–110. [CrossRef]
39. Moore, R.A.; Waheed, A.; Burns, B. *Rule of Nines*; StatPearls Publishing: Treasure Island, FL, USA, 2022.
40. Church, D.; Elsayed, S.; Reid, O.; Winston, B.; Lindsay, R. Burn Wound Infections. *Clin. Microbiol. Rev.* **2006**, *19*, 403–434. [CrossRef]
41. Hettiaratchy, S.; Papini, R. Initial management of a major burn: II—Assessment and resuscitation. *BMJ* **2004**, *329*, 101–103. [CrossRef]
42. Cirillo, M.D.; Mirdell, R.; Sjöberg, F.; Pham, T.D. Improving burn depth assessment for pediatric scalds by AI based on semantic segmentation of polarized light photography images. *Burns* **2021**, *47*, 1586–1593. [CrossRef]
43. King, A.; Balaji, S.; Keswani, S.G. Biology and Function of Fetal and Pediatric Skin. *Facial Plast. Surg. Clin. N. Am.* **2013**, *21*, 1–6. [CrossRef]
44. Lukusa, M.; Allorto, N.; Wall, S. Hypothermia in acutely presenting burn injuries to a regional burn service: The incidence and impact on outcome. *Burn. Open* **2020**, *5*, 39–44. [CrossRef]
45. Sen, S. Pediatric inhalation injury. *Burn. Trauma* **2017**, *5*, 31. [CrossRef]
46. Caruso, T.J.; Janik, L.S.; Fuzaylov, G. Airway management of recovered pediatric patients with severe head and neck burns: A review. *Pediatr. Anesth.* **2012**, *22*, 462–468. [CrossRef]
47. Nielson, C.B.; Duethman, N.C.; Howard, J.M.; Moncure, M.; Wood, J.G. Burns. *J. Burn Care Res.* **2017**, *38*, e469–e481. [CrossRef] [PubMed]
48. Strudwick, X.L.; Cowin, A.J. *The Role of the Inflammatory Response in Burn Injury*; IntechOpen: London, UK, 2017; ISBN 978-1-78923-131-1.
49. Noorbakhsh, S.I.; Bonar, E.M.; Polinski, R.; Amin, S. Educational Case: Burn Injury—Pathophysiology, Classification, and Treatment. *Acad. Pathol.* **2021**, *8*, 1–10. [CrossRef] [PubMed]
50. Singh, M.; Prakash, S. Burn: A Clinical Perspective. In *Theory and Applications of Heat Transfer in Humans*; John Wiley & Sons, Ltd.: Hoboken, NJ, USA, 2018; pp. 513–527, ISBN 978-1-119-12742-0.
51. Samuelsson, A. Effects of Burns and Vasoactive Drugs on Human Skin, Clinical and Experimental Studies Using Microdialysis. Ph.D. Thesis, Linköping University Electronic Press, Linköping, Sweden, 2022.
52. Abdulkhaleq, L.A.; Assi, M.A.; Abdullah, R.; Zamri-Saad, M.; Taufiq-Yap, Y.H.; Hezmee, M.N.M. The crucial roles of inflammatory mediators in inflammation: A review. *Vet. World* **2018**, *11*, 627–635. [CrossRef] [PubMed]

53. Mulder, P.P.G.; Vlig, M.; Boekema, B.K.H.L.; Stoop, M.M.; Pijpe, A.; van Zuijlen, P.P.M.; de Jong, E.; van Cranenbroek, B.; Joosten, I.; Koenen, H.J.P.M.; et al. Persistent Systemic Inflammation in Patients With Severe Burn Injury Is Accompanied by Influx of Immature Neutrophils and Shifts in T Cell Subsets and Cytokine Profiles. *Front. Immunol.* **2021**, *11*, 621222. [CrossRef]
54. Jeschke, M.G.; Van Baar, M.E.; Choudhry, M.A.; Chung, K.K.; Gibran, N.S.; Logsetty, S. Burn injury. *Nat. Rev. Dis. Primers* **2020**, *6*, 11. [CrossRef]
55. Evers, L.H.; Bhavsar, D.; Mailänder, P. The biology of burn injury. *Exp. Dermatol.* **2010**, *19*, 777–783. [CrossRef]
56. Korkmaz, H.I.; Ulrich, M.M.W.; van Wieringen, W.; Vlig, M.; Emmens, R.W.; Meyer, K.W.; Sinnige, P.; Krijnen, P.; van Zuijlen, P.; Niessen, H. The Local and Systemic Inflammatory Response in a Pig Burn Wound Model With a Pivotal Role for Complement. *J. Burn Care Res.* **2017**, *38*, e796–e806. [CrossRef]
57. Devine, R.; Diltz, Z.; Hall, M.W.; Thakkar, R.K. The systemic immune response to pediatric thermal injury. *Int. J. Burn. Trauma* **2018**, *8*, 6–16.
58. akir, B.; Yeğen, B.Ç. Systemic Responses to Burn Injury. *Turk. J. Med Sci.* **2004**, *34*, 215–226.
59. Toliver-Kinsky, T.; Kobayashi, M.; Suzuki, F.; Sherwood, E.R. 19—The Systemic Inflammatory Response Syndrome. In *Total Burn Care*, 5th ed.; Herndon, D.N., Ed.; Elsevier: Amsterdam, The Netherlands, 2018; pp. 205–220.e4, ISBN 978-0-323-47661-4.
60. Keller, S. Metabolic Effects of Cytokines in Burns Trauma and Sepsis—Wound Healing. Available online: https://www.alpfmedical.info/wound-healing/metabolic-effects-of-cytokines-in-burns-trauma-and-sepsis.html (accessed on 21 February 2022).
61. Sojka, J.; Krakowski, A.C.; Stawicki, S.P. *Burn Shock and Resuscitation: Many Priorities, One Goal*; Intechopen: London, UK, 2020. [CrossRef]
62. Schaefer, T.J.; Nunez Lopez, O. *Burn Resuscitation and Management*; StatPearls Publishing: Treasure Island, FL, USA, 2022.
63. Rae, L.; Fidler, P.; Gibran, N. The Physiologic Basis of Burn Shock and the Need for Aggressive Fluid Resuscitation. *Crit. Care Clin.* **2016**, *32*, 491–505. [CrossRef]
64. Bittner, M.E.A.; Shank, M.E.; Woodson, L.C.; Martyn, M.J.A.J. Acute and Perioperative Care of the Burn-injured Patient. *Anesthesiology* **2015**, *122*, 448–464. [CrossRef]
65. Romanowski, K.S.; Palmieri, T.L. Pediatric burn resuscitation: Past, present, and future. *Burn. Trauma* **2017**, *5*, 26. [CrossRef]
66. Sharma, R.K.; Parashar, A. Special considerations in paediatric burn patients. *Indian J. Plast. Surg.* **2010**, *43*, 43–50. [CrossRef]
67. Wurzer, P.; Culnan, D.; Cancio, L.C.; Kramer, G.C. Pathophysiology of Burn Shock and Burn Edema. In *Total Burn Care*, 5th ed.; Elsevier: Amsterdam, The Netherlands, 2018; pp. 66–76.e3. [CrossRef]
68. Causbie, J.M.; Sattler, L.A.; Basel, A.P.; Britton, G.W.; Cancio, L.C. State of the Art: An Update on Adult Burn Resuscitation. *Eur. Burn J.* **2021**, *2*, 12. [CrossRef]
69. Kara, Y.A. *Burn Etiology and Pathogenesis*; IntechOpen: London, UK, 2018; ISBN 978-1-78923-131-1.
70. Williams, F.N.; Herndon, D.N.; Suman, O.E.; Lee, J.O.; Norbury, W.B.; Branski, L.K.; Mlcak, R.P.; Jeschke, M.G. Changes in Cardiac Physiology After Severe Burn Injury. *J. Burn Care Res.* **2011**, *32*, 269–274. [CrossRef]
71. Dash, S.; Ghosh, S. Transient Diabetes Insipidus Following Thermal Burn—A Case Report and Literature Review. *Bull. Emerg. Trauma* **2017**, *5*, 311–313. [CrossRef]
72. Ciftci, A.; Esen, O.; Yazicioglu, M.B.; Haksal, M.C.; Tiryaki, C.; Gunes, A.; Civil, O.; Ozyildiz, M.; Esen, H.; Ciftci, A.; et al. Could Neutrophil-to-Lymphocyte Ratio Be a New Mortality Predictor Value in Severe Burns? *J. Surg. Surg. Res.* **2019**, *5*, 026–028.
73. Andreu-Ballester, J.C.; Pons-Castillo, A.; González-Sánchez, A.; Llombart-Cussac, A.; Cano, M.J.; Cuéllar, C. Lymphopenia in hospitalized patients and its relationship with severity of illness and mortality. *PLoS ONE* **2021**, *16*, e0256205. [CrossRef]
74. Singh, V.; Devgan, L.; Bhat, S.; Milner, S.M. The Pathogenesis of Burn Wound Conversion. *Ann. Plast. Surg.* **2007**, *59*, 109–115. [CrossRef]
75. Mariano, F.; de Biase, C.; Hollo, Z.; Deambrosis, I.; Davit, A.; Mella, A.; Bergamo, D.; Maffei, S.; Rumbolo, F.; Papaleo, A.; et al. Long-Term Preservation of Renal Function in Septic Shock Burn Patients Requiring Renal Replacement Therapy for Acute Kidney Injury. *J. Clin. Med.* **2021**, *10*, 5760. [CrossRef]
76. Lang, T.C.; Zhao, R.; Kim, A.; Wijewardena, A.; Vandervord, J.; Xue, M.; Jackson, C.J. A Critical Update of the Assessment and Acute Management of Patients with Severe Burns. *Adv. Wound Care* **2019**, *8*, 607–633. [CrossRef]
77. Sobouti, B.; Fallah, S.; Ghavami, Y.; Moradi, M. Serum immunoglobulin levels in pediatric burn patients. *Burns* **2013**, *39*, 473–476. [CrossRef]
78. Megha, K.B.; Mohanan, P.V. Role of immunoglobulin and antibodies in disease management. *Int. J. Biol. Macromol.* **2020**, *169*, 28–38. [CrossRef]
79. Boldeanu, L.; Boldeanu, M.V.; Bogdan, M.; Meca, A.D.; Coman, C.G.; Buca, B.R.; Tartau, C.G.; Tartau, L.M. Immunological approaches and therapy in burns (Review). *Exp. Ther. Med.* **2020**, *20*, 2361–2367. [CrossRef]
80. Yussof, S.J.M.; Omar, E.; Pai, D.; Sood, S. Cellular events and biomarkers of wound healing. *Indian J. Plast. Surg.* **2012**, *45*, 220–228. [CrossRef]
81. Strbo, N.; Yin, N.; Stojadinovic, O. Innate and Adaptive Immune Responses in Wound Epithelialization. *Adv. Wound Care* **2014**, *3*, 492–501. [CrossRef]
82. Ellis, S.; Lin, E.J.; Tartar, D. Immunology of Wound Healing. *Curr. Dermatol. Rep.* **2018**, *7*, 350–358. [CrossRef]
83. Suda, S.; Williams, H.; Medbury, H.J.; Holland, A.J.A. A Review of Monocytes and Monocyte-Derived Cells in Hypertrophic Scarring Post Burn. *J. Burn Care Res.* **2016**, *37*, 265–272. [CrossRef]

84. Beckmann, N.; Schumacher, F.; Kleuser, B.; Gulbins, E.; Nomellini, V.; Caldwell, C.C. Burn Injury Impairs Neutrophil Chemotaxis through Increased Ceramide. *Shock* **2020**, *56*, 125–132. [CrossRef]
85. Jiang, Y.; Chen, M.; Nie, H.; Yuan, Y. PD-1 and PD-L1 in cancer immunotherapy: Clinical implications and future considerations. *Hum. Vaccines Immunother.* **2019**, *15*, 1111–1122. [CrossRef]
86. Grywalska, E.; Smarz-Widelska, I.; Korona-Głowniak, I.; Mertowski, S.; Gosik, K.; Hymos, A.; Ludian, J.; Niedźwiedzka-Rystwej, P.; Roliński, J.; Załuska, W. PD-1 and PD-L1 Expression on Circulating Lymphocytes as a Marker of Epstein-Barr Virus Reactivation-Associated Proliferative Glomerulonephritis. *Int. J. Mol. Sci.* **2020**, *21*, 8001. [CrossRef] [PubMed]
87. Van Coillie, S.; Wiernicki, B.; Xu, J. Molecular and Cellular Functions of CTLA-4. In *Regulation of Cancer Immune Checkpoints: Molecular and Cellular Mechanisms and Therapy*; Xu, J., Ed.; Advances in Experimental Medicine and Biology; Springer: Singapore, 2020; pp. 7–32, ISBN 9789811532665.

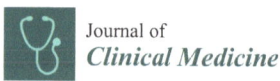 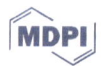

Article

Clinical Evaluation of the Efficacy and Tolerability of Rigenase® and Polyhexanide (Fitostimoline® Plus) vs. Hyaluronic Acid and Silver Sulfadiazine (Connettivina® Bio Plus) for the Treatment of Acute Skin Wounds: A Randomized Trial

Raffaele Russo [1], Albino Carrizzo [1,2], Alfonso Barbato [3], Barbara Rosa Rasile [1], Paola Pentangelo [1], Alessandra Ceccaroni [1], Caterina Marra [1], Carmine Alfano [1,*] and Luigi Losco [1,*]

[1] Plastic Surgery Unit, Department of Medicine, Surgery and Dentistry, University of Salerno, Baronissi, 84081 Salerno, Italy; rafrusso@unisa.it (R.R.); acarrizzo@unisa.it (A.C.); barbara.rasile@gmail.com (B.R.R.); paolapentangelo1995@gmail.com (P.P.); aceccaroni@unisa.it (A.C.); camarra@unisa.it (C.M.)
[2] Vascular Physiopathology Unit, IRCCS Neuromed, 86077 Pozzilli, Italy
[3] U.O.C. di Chirurgia Plastica Ricostruttiva, Azienda Ospedaliera Universitaria OO.RR. San Giovanni di Dio e Ruggi d'Aragona, Via S. Leonardo 1, 84131 Salerno, Italy; alfonso.barbato@sangiovannieruggi.it
* Correspondence: calfano@unisa.it (C.A.); luigi.losco@gmail.com (L.L.)

Abstract: Objectives: Compare the efficacy and tolerability of Connettivina® Bio Plus (Group A) gauze and cream, and Fitostimoline® Plus (Group B) gauze and cream for the treatment of acute superficial skin lesions. Design: Single-center, parallel, randomized trial. A block randomization method was used. Setting: University of Salerno—AOU San Giovanni di Dio e Ruggi d'Aragona. Participants: Sixty patients were enrolled. All patients fulfilled the study requirements. Intervention: One application of the study drugs every 24 h, and a six-week observation period. Main outcome measures: Efficacy and tolerability of the study drugs. Results: In total, 60 patients (Group A, $n = 30$; Group B, $n = 30$) were randomized; mean age was 58.5 ± 15.8 years. All patients were included in the outcome analysis. Total wound healing was achieved in 17 patients undergoing treatment with Connettivina® Bio Plus and 28 patients undergoing treatment with Fitostimoline® Plus. The greater effectiveness of the latter was significant ($p = 0.00104$). In Group B, a significantly greater degree of effectiveness was observed in reducing the fibrin in the wound bed ($p = 0.04746$). Complications or unexpected events were not observed. Conclusions: Both Connettivina® Bio Plus and Fitostimoline® Plus are secure and effective for treating acute superficial skin lesions. Fitostimoline® Plus was more effective than Connettivina® Bio Plus in wound healing of acute superficial skin lesions, especially if fibrin had been observed in the wound bed.

Keywords: wound healing; acute skin wound; hyaluronic acid; aqueous extract of *Triticum vulgare*; TVE; Rigenase; Connettivina Bio Plus; Fitostimoline Plus; randomized trial

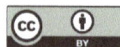

1. Introduction

Nowadays, health care professionals are frequently called upon to manage acute or chronic wounds; their management may often lead to complications representing a "silent epidemic" [1]. A deep knowledge of the complex synchronized cascade involved in the anatomical and functional integrity of the skin is essential; on the other hand, methods and materials for wound management should be well acknowledged [2–5]. Timely treatment of acute skin lesions is paramount to prevent delayed wound healing, chronicization of the wound, and subsequent increases in health care costs [6].

Hyaluronic acid (HA) is a major component of the extracellular matrix (ECM) of the skin, joints, and many other tissues [7]. Owing to its remarkable biomedical and tissue regeneration potential, HA is widely employed in modern medicine under different formulations such as gauzes, fillers, injective, creams, and gels. It shows a wide range of pharmacological activities, including anti-inflammatory [8], wound-healing and tissue-regenerating [9–11], immunomodulatory [12], and cosmetic properties [13]. HA is involved in each phase of wound healing: it stimulates cell migration, differentiation, and proliferation; moreover, it regulates ECM organization and metabolism. HA was combined with silver sulfadiazine (SSD), which prevents colonization of the wound [14], to create an advanced dressing marketed under the brand name Connettivina® Bio Plus gauzes and cream (Fidia Farmaceutici S.p.A., Abano Terme, Italy).

Rigenase® is a specific extract of *Triticum vulgare* (TVE); it retains a scavenger effect against free radicals, thus showing significant antioxidant activity. It also maximizes the tissue regeneration process through an increase in chemotaxis, fibroblastic proliferation, and maturation. These properties are due to the increase in protein synthesis, proline uptake, and the upregulation of many fundamental factors such as MMP-2, MMP-9, collagen I, and elastin [15]. It is used to treat pressure sores, venous leg ulcers, wounds, burns, delays in scarring, dystrophic conditions, and, more generally, problems related to re-epithelialization or tissue regeneration [16]. Rigenase® was combined with poliesanide (PHMB), which prevents colonization and contamination of the wound [17], to create the medical device Fitostimoline® Plus gauzes and cream (Farmaceutici Damor S.p.A., Napoli, Italy).

Fitostimoline® Plus and Connettivina® Bio Plus are widely used, and they are both considered effective treatments of acute and chronic skin lesions; however, to the best of our knowledge, they have never been compared for the treatment of acute skin lesions. The aim of our study was to compare the efficacy and tolerability of two advanced dressings for the treatment of acute superficial skin lesions.

2. Patients and Methods

This was a single-center, equally randomized (1:1), parallel group study conducted at the University of Salerno, AOU San Giovanni di Dio e Ruggi d'Aragona, from September 2020 to December 2021. Eligible patients were all adults above 18 years of age and presenting with an acute skin lesion related to burn, trauma, or surgical wound dehiscence.

Patients with any of the following conditions were excluded from study participation: pregnancy or breastfeeding; inadequate contraceptive procedures in fertile women; chronic concomitant treatment with local antiseptics, use of anti-inflammatory (steroid and non-steroidal), analgesic, antineoplastic, or immunosuppressive drugs; non-therapeutic use of psychoactive substances; abuse of drugs and/or alcohol; immunodeficiencies (i.e., HIV infection); current neoplastic diseases; known allergies, hypersensitivity, or intolerance to any of the substances administered in this trial; any medical or non-medical condition which could significantly reduce the possibility of obtaining reliable data and achieve the objectives of the study; any condition that may affect the validity of the informed consent and/or compromise the patient's adherence to the study procedures; treatment with any study dressings in the last 30 days prior to the start of the study; a previous enrollment in this study.

According to the results of a pilot study conducted in our University Hospital, healing was expected in 90% of patients treated with Fitostimoline® Plus (Farmaceutici Damor S.p.A., Napoli, Italy), versus 60% of patients treated with Connettivina® Bio Plus (Fidia Farmaceutici S.p.A., Abano Terme, Italy). Relying on this assumption, the data of 29 patients per group should be analyzed to obtain a power of 80% and a two-sided 5% significance level. Given an anticipated dropout rate of 5%, 60 patients should be enrolled (30 per group).

2.1. Treatment Plan

Sixty patients complying with the admission criteria were included in the study, and randomly assigned to receive either Connettivina® Bio Plus (Fidia Farmaceutici S.p.A., Abano Terme, Italy) in the form of cream and gauze, or Fitostimoline® Plus (Farmaceutici Damor S.p.A., Napoli, Italy) in the form of cream and gauze. A block randomization was generated using a computer and prepared by an investigator with no clinical involvement in the study. Informed consent was obtained from a member of the medical staff, and the physician made a phone call to an investigator who was independent of the recruitment process to assign participants to interventions.

The study plan included a six-week observation period; it was organized as follows: on the baseline visit (V1), randomization was accomplished, and after proper information, informed consent was signed. Patients assigned to Group A (Connettivina® Bio Plus Fidia Farmaceutici S.p.A., Abano Terme, Italy) were treated as follows: Connettivina® Bio Plus cream (Fidia Farmaceutici S.p.A., Abano Terme, Italy), one application every 24 h; Connettivina® Bio Plus gauze (Fidia Farmaceutici S.p.A., Abano Terme, Italy), one application every 24 h. Patients assigned to Group B (Fitostimoline® Plus) were treated as follows: Fitostimoline® Plus cream (Farmaceutici Damor S.p.A., Napoli, Italy), one application every 24 h; Fitostimoline® Plus gauze (Farmaceutici Damor S.p.A., Napoli, Italy), one application every 24 h. Wound dressing was performed as follows: the wound bed was uniformly covered with cream, then soaked gauzes were applied and covered with a sterile gauze; bandaging was performed if necessary. If needed, a surgical debridement was performed by the Principal Investigator (C.A.) at the clinic before the baseline visit. Follow-up visits were scheduled every 7 ± 1 days (V2, V3, V4, and V5), and the final visit (V6) was planned after 45 ± 2 days. The number of planned visits could be lower than previously stated in the case of healing or withdrawal from the study. An unplanned visit could be held if required by the patient. During V1, the informed consent was signed, and personal data (age, weight and height, medical history, vital parameters, and ongoing drug therapies) were collected; a picture of the lesion was taken. At the intermediate visits and at the last visit (V2–V6), eventual therapy changes, vital parameters, and the evaluation of eventual side effects were investigated. During every visit, a physical examination of the wound and the assessment of related symptoms were performed; moreover, the evaluation of wound edges and perilesional area was carried out. The physical exam of the wound, including location and size, the presence of fibrin, granulation tissue, infection, and maceration of the wound edges, was evaluated too. The physical exam of the wound edges (defined as the external margins of the lesion) included the assessment of erythema, bleeding, pain, burn, and itch; each of them was scored on a scale of 0 to 3 (0 = absent, 1 = mild, 2 = moderate, and 3 = severe). The physical exam of perilesional skin (the skin immediately adjacent to the wound edges) included the assessment of erythema, edema, pain, burn, itch, and dryness; the score system was the same as previously described. All the scores were summed to obtain the Total Symptoms Score (TSS); this was calculated for both the wound edges and perilesional skin. From V2 onwards, tolerability and adherence to the treatment were considered, and in the case of any systemic or local adverse event, patient withdrawal from the study was mandatory (Table 1).

Table 1. Study design.

	V1	V2	V3	V4	V5	V6
Informed consent	•					
Evaluation of admission criteria	•	•	•	•	•	•
Randomization	•					
Demographical data	•					
Anamnestic data	•					
Associated therapies	•	•	•	•	•	•
Vitals (BP, BPM, T) [1]	•	•	•	•	•	•
Clinical examination of the lesion	•	•	•	•	•	•
Planimetry of lesion	•	•	•	•	•	•
Side effects		•	•	•	•	•

[1] BP, Blood Pressure; BPM, Beats per Minute; T, Temperature.

The trial adhered to established procedures to maintain separation between staff that took outcome measurements and staff that delivered the intervention.

2.2. Endpoints

Primary endpoint: The main goal of this study was the evaluation of the efficacy of HA and silver sulfadiazine in the form of soaked gauzes and cream, compared to Rigenase® and polyhexanide in the same forms. The assessment was based on the wound healing rate (WHR), evaluated as the rate of the reduction in the wound area when compared to the baseline visit (V1). Total wound healing was considered as the complete healing of the acute lesion assessed in V6 or during an earlier visit; partial wound healing was considered as incomplete healing achieved in V6.

Secondary endpoints: The evolution of the wound edges and perilesional skin was based on signs and symptoms, and these were evaluated according to the Total Symptoms Score (TSS). The tolerability of both study drugs was assessed. The schematic flowchart of the study is presented in Figure 1.

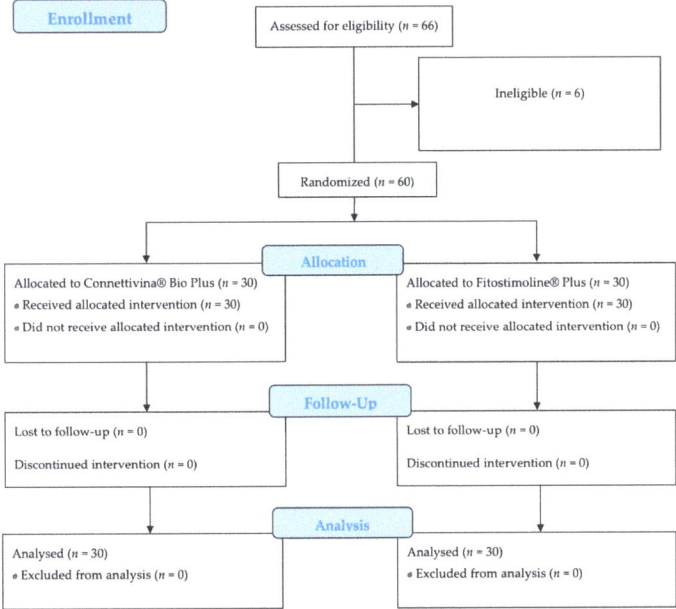

Figure 1. Schematic flowchart of the study.

2.3. Statistical Analysis

Statistical analysis was performed using SPSS Statistics software package version 25 (IBM Corp. SPSS Statistics for Windows, New York, NY, USA). Parametric data were provided as mean ± standard deviation and range. The homogeneity of the study groups was evaluated using the two-tailed Mann–Whitney test, Chi-squared, Z-test, and the Kruskal–Wallis test. The primary endpoint was investigated using the Z-test and the Kruskal–Wallis test. The secondary endpoint was investigated using the two-tailed Mann–Whitney test. The significance was set at a value of $p < 0.05$.

3. Results

Sixty patients affected with acute superficial skin lesions of any origin were recruited and randomly assigned to a treatment group (Group A, $n = 30$; Group B, $n = 30$). Six patients were excluded due to ineligibility.

The average age of the patients was 58.5 ± 15.8 years. The average number of days elapsed between V1 and complete healing or V6 was 42.3 ± 6.2 days in Group A and 35.4 ± 8.2 days in Group B (Table 2).

Table 2. Patients and treatments.

Variable	Value	
Patients	60	
Age, years	58.5 ± 15.8	
Gender, female	28 (46.6%)	
	Group A	Group B
Days of treatment (until healing or V6)	42.3 ± 6.2	35.4 ± 8.2
Acute skin wounds		
Surgical wound	19 (63.3%)	14 (46%)
Burn	2 (6.6%)	5 (16.6%)
Trauma	9 (30%)	11 (36.6%)

Group A. Connettivina® Bio Plus; Group B. Fitostimoline® Plus.

As shown in Table 3, there were no significant differences between the two groups in terms of age, sex, area of the skin lesion assessed at V1(baseline), and wound etiology. The mean lesion area progressively decreased from baseline to V6. Both treatment protocols were effective ($p < 0.001$) (Figure 2) (Table 3).

Table 3. Differences in gender, age, wound area, and wound etiology between the populations under exam.

	Group A	Group B	p
Gender, m	16	15	0.79
Age, years	57.1 ± 14.1	59.9 ± 17.5	0.14
Wound area (V1), cm^2	25.9 ± 20.8	32.1 ± 21.4	>0.99
Wound etiology			
Surgical wound	19	14	0.19
Burn	2	5	0.22
Trauma	9	11	0.58

Group A, Connettivina® Bio Plus; Group B, Fitostimoline® Plus.

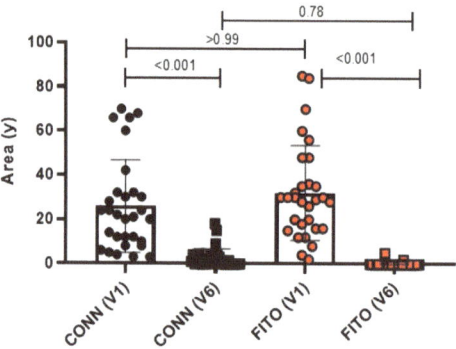

Figure 2. Effectiveness of treatment protocols. Conn(v1), wound area in patients treated with Connettivina® Bio Plus in V1; Conn (V6), wound area in patients treated with Connettivina® Bio Plus in V6; Fito(v1), wound area in patients treated with Fitostimoline® Plus in V1; Fito (V6), wound area in patients treated with Fitostimoline® Plus in V6.

Total wound healing was achieved in 17 patients undergoing treatment with Connettivina® Bio Plus, and in 28 patients undergoing treatment with Fitostimoline® Plus. The greater effectiveness of Fitostimoline® Plus was significant ($p = 0.001$, risk ratio 0.15 (95% CI 0.04 to 0.62)). The reduction in the wound area was assessed. The wound healing rate was greater in Group B; however, these data were not statistically significant. A reduction in fibrin and maceration of the wound edges was observed in both treatment groups; however, Group B showed more satisfying results regarding reduction of fibrin on the wound bed ($p = 0.04$, risk ratio 0.2 (95% CI 0.02 to 1.70)) (Table 4) (Figures 3 and 4).

Table 4. Treatment and outcomes.

Outcome	Group A	Group B	p-Value	Risk Ratio (95% CI)
Total wound healing, patients	56.6% (17)	93.3% (28)	0.001	0.15 (0.04 to 0.62)
Wound area, cm²	V1: 25.9 ± 20.8 [95% CI 18.1 to 33.6] V6: 2.4 ± 4.4 [95% CI 0.8 to 4.1]	V1: 32.1 ± 21.4 [95% CI 24.1 to 40.1] V6: 0.2 ± 1.0 [95% CI −0.13 to 0.6]	0.78	
Fibrin on wound bed, healed patients	77% (10)	95% (21)	0.04	0.2 (0.02 to 1.70)
Maceration of wound edges, healed patients	100% (6)	100% (7)	0.90	0.88 (0.02 to 38.59)

Group A, Connettivina® Bio Plus; Group B, Fitostimoline® Plus.

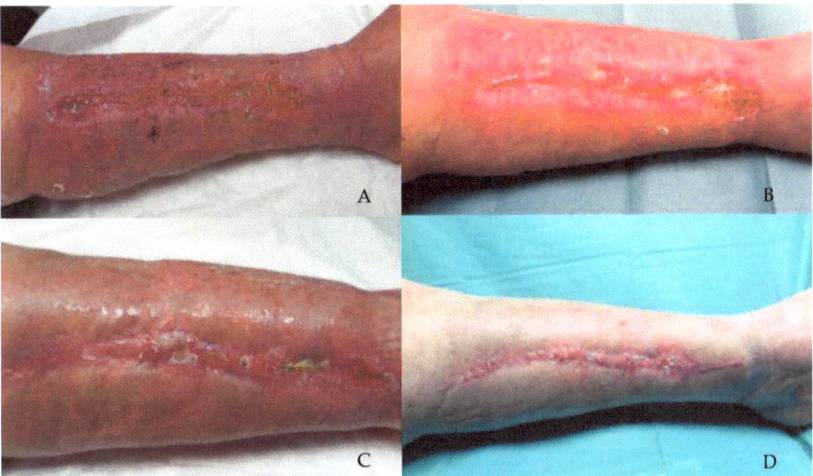

Figure 3. A 75-year-old female patient presented with a wound dehiscence localized on the medial aspect of the left leg. The patient was randomly assigned to the group treated with Connettivina® Bio Plus cream and gauze. (**A**) Patient in V1. Wound bed is partially covered with fibrin, wound borders and perilesional skin are erythematous, and edema is observed. (**B**) Wound in V3, wound area sensibly reduced, wound bed exudate decreased considerably, although fibrin remained. Perilesional skin and wound borders improved overall. (**C**) Wound in V5. (**D**) V6, wound completely healed, and perilesional skin was a physiologic color.

Wound edges and perilesional skin TSS reduction was evaluated, and no statistical difference was observed between the study groups, $p = 0.28$ and $p = 0.99$, respectively. The TSS is a good clinical method for following the improvement related to a specific patient; however, some of the domains are merely subjective, and this could be a limitation of this evaluation method.

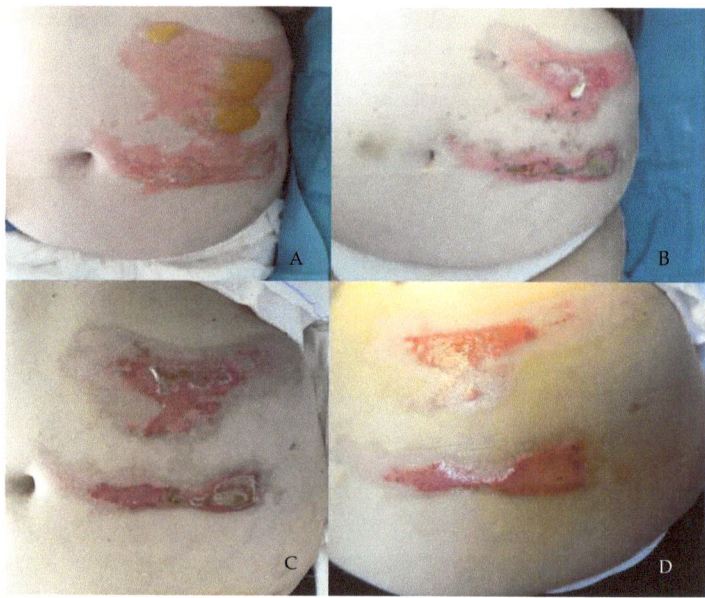

Figure 4. A 69-year-old female patient presented with a first- and second-degree burn lesion localized on the left side of the abdomen. The patient was randomly assigned to the group treated with Fitostimoline® Plus cream and gauze. (**A**) Patient in V1, wound bed is covered with blisters; wound borders and perilesional skin are erythematous and edematous. (**B**) Patient in V3, wound area sensibly lessened (first-degree burn lesion); fibrin could be detected on the wound bed. Edema and erythema subsided significantly. (**C**) Wound in V5. (**D**) V6, wound healed completely.

4. Discussion

Acute superficial skin lesions arising after burns, traumas, or as a complication of surgical procedures are major concerns [18–21]. These lesions could be challenging, especially in older and complex patients, if lower limbs are involved, or if an infection occurs [22–24]. When an acute skin injury occurs, the ECM array is altered in association with other mediators, and HA helps with maintaining the structural integrity of the skin; moreover, it creates a favorable environment for fibroblasts, which lead the way to develop proper granulating tissue [25]. HA was conjugated with SSD to create the advanced dressing known as Connettivina® Bio Plus. This combination helps to prevent one of the downsides of SSD, which is delayed wound healing. Although the exact mechanism is yet to be fully understood, some data suggest that SSD impairs the cytokine milieu that results in aberrant recruitment and the activation of macrophages [26]. However, SSD retains a relevant bactericidal effect: through the impairment of DNA replication, it generates an increase in cell-wall permeability and the formation of free radicals [27].

Rigenase®, on the other hand, shows excellent skin repair properties. This plant-derived polysaccharide has the ability to induce the biosynthesis and release of specific proteins from keratinocytes. The majority of these secreted proteins are effectors in cell cross-talk and are involved in tissue repair and regeneration. In particular, Rigenase® favors cell migration and stimulates the synthesis of new ECM [28–30]. The cationic polymer polyhexanide, an active factor in Fitostimoline® Plus, interferes with the stability of bacterial cell membrane binding to anionic phospholipids. At the same time, its interaction with human cells is very limited, making the risk–benefit ratio superior to other antimicrobial agents [31]. Soaked gauzes and cream formulations of Connettivina® Bio Plus and Fitostimoline® Plus are frequently used, not only for the treatment of acute skin lesions, but also chronic wounds, burns, and pressure sores. Moreover, these are often used as dressings of skin flaps and skin grafts following reconstructive surgery [32–35] and could be used with negative pressure treatments [36,37]. Costagliola et al. [38] showed that HA formulations were effective and well tolerated for the treatment of second-degree burns. It was also demonstrated that HA-based products could enhance healing following surgery or laser skin resurfacing [14,39]. Martini et al. [40] investigated the effects of two different formulations of TVE (soaked gauzes and cream) in comparison to a gel form of equine catalase (Citrizan) for the topical treatment of small-to-medium-sized second-degree burns. The authors found that the healing rates of burn lesions and re-epithelialization >95% were higher in the Fitostimoline® soaked gauzes and gel-pooled groups than in the Catalase gel group. To the best of our knowledge, the efficacy and tolerability of Connettivina® Bio Plus and Fitostimoline® Plus have never been compared for the treatment of acute superficial skin lesions. In the present study, every patient was randomly assigned to a treatment group. Seventeen patients in the group (A) and twenty-eight patients in the group (B) recovered completely. A greater reduction in the wound area was observed in Group B; however, these data were not statistically significant, probably due to the low numbers of the cohorts in exam; nevertheless, this is the first study comparing both medications, and there are no similar studies with a larger number of patients. Both the treatment drugs were effective in reducing the fibrin within the lesion; however, in Group B, significant major effectiveness was observed. These findings are consistent with the current literature: it is widely demonstrated that a reduction in fibrin promotes the removal of corrupted matrix and stimulates the accumulation of a competent provisional matrix, thus facilitating a physiological healing process [41–43]. Data available from the literature about improvement in signs and symptoms after treatment with either TVE or HA are limited. HA showed pain-relieving activity in osteoarthritis patients and for periodontitis [44]. Cellular oxidative stress plays a significant role in burn symptoms; consequently, the antioxidant activity of Fitostimoline® Plus may be a key factor that either blocks or scavenges free radical generation in inflammatory tissue [45]. According to the literature, HA presents an excellent reduction in burning sensation [46]; erythema could be downgraded by both HA and TVE [47–49]. The TSS is a good clinical method to follow improvement related to a specific patient. However, some of the domains are merely subjective, and this could be a limitation of this evaluation method. The sample size, although conspicuous, is a limitation of the present study. The aim of our study was to assess the effectiveness of Rigenase® and HA for the treatment of the most common acute superficial skin lesions, including burn, traumatic wound, or surgical wound dehiscence. The disarray of ECM and the need for a firm approach for fast recovery are major common points. We are aware that even though the pathological mechanisms in burn and surgical wounds differ [50,51], the skin biomechanics and reepithelization could be comparable, and for this reason, we chose to include all of them in our study. The frequency of each type of wound (burn, post-surgical, and traumatic) was tested to exclude any statistically significant difference between the two treatment groups. However, a prospective, multicenter study that evaluates treatment outcomes of a single specific type of wound (i.e., burn) should be advocated. The results of the present trial could help with designing future studies, and physicians that are called to manage acute skin wounds could be aided by our findings.

5. Conclusions

Both Connettivina® Bio Plus and Fitostimoline® Plus are secure and effective for the treatment of acute superficial skin lesions. Fitostimoline® Plus was proven to be more effective than Connettivina® Bio Plus in healing acute superficial skin lesions; moreover, it was more effective in wound healing if fibrin had been observed in the wound bed.

Author Contributions: Conceptualization, A.C. (Albino Carrizzo), A.B., C.A., and L.L.; methodology, R.R., A.C. (Albino Carrizzo), A.C. (Alessandra Ceccaroni), C.M., and L.L.; software, R.R., A.C. (Albino Carrizzo), B.R.R., and P.P.; validation, C.A. and L.L.; formal analysis, A.C. (Albino Carrizzo), A.B., B.R.R., A.C. (Alessandra Ceccaroni), C.M., and L.L.; investigation, P.P., A.C. (Alessandra Ceccaroni), C.M., and L.L.; resources, R.R., A.C. (Albino Carrizzo), A.B., C.A., and L.L.; data curation, R.R., A.C. (Albino Carrizzo), A.C. (Alessandra Ceccaroni), C.M., and L.L.; writing—original draft preparation, B.R.R., P.P., A.C. (Alessandra Ceccaroni), C.M., and L.L.; writing—review and editing, R.R., A.B., C.A., and L.L.; visualization, R.R., A.C. (Albino Carrizzo), C.A., and L.L.; supervision, A.B., C.A., and L.L.; project administration, C.A. and L.L. All authors have read and agreed to the published version of the manuscript.

Funding: This research received no external funding.

Institutional Review Board Statement: The study was conducted in accordance with the Declaration of Helsinki and approved by the Institutional Review Board Campania Sud (Nr 0138589).

Informed Consent Statement: Informed consent was obtained from all subjects involved in the study.

Data Availability Statement: The data presented in this study are available on request from the corresponding author C.A. The data are not publicly available due to privacy restrictions.

Conflicts of Interest: The authors declare no conflict of interest.

References

1. Järbrink, K.; Ni, G.; Sönnergren, H.; Schmidtchen, A.; Pang, C.; Bajpai, R.; Car, J. Prevalence and incidence of chronic wounds and related complications: A protocol for a systematic review. *Syst. Rev.* **2016**, *5*, 152. [CrossRef] [PubMed]
2. Martin, J.M.; Zenilman, J.M.; Lazarus, G.S. Molecular microbiology: New dimensions for cutaneous biology and wound healing. *J. Investig. Dermatol.* **2010**, *130*, 38–48. [CrossRef]
3. Marcasciano, M.; Kaciulyte, J.; Mori, F.L.R.; Lo Torto, F.; Barellini, L.; Loreti, A.; Fanelli, B.; De Vita, R.; Redi, U.; Marcasciano, F.; et al. Breast surgeons updating on the thresholds of COVID-19 era: Results of a multicenter collaborative study evaluating the role of online videos and multimedia sources on breast surgeons education and training. *Eur. Rev. Med. Pharmacol. Sci.* **2020**, *24*, 7845–7854. [CrossRef] [PubMed]
4. Menichini, G.; Alfano, C.; Provenzano, E.; Marrelli, M.; Statti, G.A.; Conforti, F. Cachrys pungens Jan inhibits human melanoma cell proliferation through photo-induced cytotoxic activity. *Cell Prolif.* **2012**, *45*, 39–47. [CrossRef] [PubMed]
5. Ciacci, C.; Globularia Alypum, L. Modulates Inflammatory Markers in the Human Colon and shows a Potential Antioxidant Role in Myeloid Leukemic Cells. *Transl. Med. UniSa* **2022**, *24*, 4. [CrossRef]
6. Cigna, E.; Pierazzi, D.M.; Sereni, S.; Marcasciano, M.; Losco, L.; Bolletta, A. Lymphatico-venous anastomosis in chronic ulcer with venous insufficiency: A case report. *Microsurgery* **2021**, *41*, 574–578. [CrossRef]
7. Vasvani, S.; Kulkarni, P.; Rawtani, D. Hyaluronic acid: A review on its biology, aspects of drug delivery, route of administrations and a special emphasis on its approved marketed products and recent clinical studies. *Int. J. Biol. Macromol.* **2020**, *151*, 1012–1029. [CrossRef]
8. Litwiniuk, M.; Krejner, A.; Speyrer, M.S.; Gauto, A.R.; Grzela, T. Hyaluronic Acid in Inflammation and Tissue Regeneration. *Wounds* **2016**, *28*, 78–88.
9. Jiang, D.; Liang, J.; Noble, P.W. Hyaluronan as an immune regulator in human diseases. *Physiol. Rev.* **2011**, *91*, 221–264. [CrossRef]
10. Lo Torto, F.; Redi, U.; Cigna, E.; Losco, L.; Marcasciano, M.; Casella, D.; Ciudad, P.; Ribuffo, D. Nasal Reconstruction with Two Stages Versus Three Stages Forehead Fap: What is Better for Patients with High Vascular Risk? *J. Craniofacial Surg.* **2020**, *31*, e57–e60. [CrossRef]
11. Marcasciano, M.; Mazzocchi, M.; Kaciulyte, J.; Spissu, N.; Casella, D.; Ribuffo, D.; Dessy, L.A. Skin cancers and dermal substitutes: Is it safe? Review of the literature and presentation of a 2-stage surgical protocol for the treatment of non-melanoma skin cancers of the head in fragile patients. *Int. Wound J.* **2018**, *15*, 756–768. [CrossRef] [PubMed]
12. Weiss, L.; Slavin, S.; Reich, S.; Cohen, P.; Shuster, S.; Stern, R.; Kaganovsky, E.; Okon, E.; Rubinstein, A.M.; Naor, D. Induction of resistance to diabetes in non-obese diabetic mice by targeting CD44 with a specific monoclonal antibody. *Proc. Natl. Acad. Sci. USA* **2000**, *97*, 285–290. [CrossRef] [PubMed]
13. Olczyk, P.; Komosińska-Vassev, K.; Winsz-Szczotka, K.; Kuźnik-Trocha, K.; Olczyk, K. Hialuronian–struktura, metabolizm, funkcje i rola w procesach gojenia ran [Hyaluronan: Structure, metabolism, functions, and role in wound healing]. *Postepy Hig. Med. Dosw* **2008**, *62*, 651–659. (In Polish)
14. Kontoes, P.P.; Vrettou, C.P.; Loupatatzi, A.N.; Marayiannis, K.V.; Foukas, P.G.; Vlachos, S.P. Wound healing after laser skin resurfacing: The effect of a silver sulfadiazine-hyaluronic acid-containing cream under an occlusive dressing. *J. Cosmet. Laser Ther.* **2010**, *12*, 10–13. [CrossRef]
15. Antonucci, I.; Fiorentino, G.; Contursi, P.; Minale, M.; Riccio, R.; Riccio, S.; Limauro, D. Antioxidant Capacity of Rigenase®, a Specific Aqueous Extract of Triticum vulgare. *Antioxidants* **2018**, *7*, 67. [CrossRef]

16. Kramer, A.; Dissemond, J.; Kim, S.; Willy, C.; Mayer, D.; Papke, R.; Tuchmann, F.; Assadian, O. Consensus on Wound Antisepsis: Update 2018. *Skin Pharmacol. Physiol.* **2018**, *31*, 28–58. [CrossRef]
17. Koburger, T.; Hubner, N.O.; Braun, M.; Siebert, J.; Kramer, A. Standardized comparison of antiseptic efficacy of triclosan, PVP-iodine, octenidine dihydrochloride, polyhexanide and chlorhexidine digluconate. *J. Antimicrob. Chemother.* **2010**, *65*, 1712–1719. [CrossRef]
18. Losco, L.; Lo Torto, F.; Maruccia, M.; Di Taranto, G.; Ribuffo, D.; Cigna, E. Modified single pedicle reverse adipofascial flap for fingertip reconstruction. *Microsurgery* **2019**, *39*, 221–227. [CrossRef]
19. Losco, L.; Cigna, E. Aesthetic Refinements in C-V Flap: Raising a Perfect Cylinder. *Aesthetic Surg. J.* **2018**, *38*, NP26–NP28. [CrossRef]
20. Kaddoura, I.; Abu-Sittah, G.; Ibrahim, A.; Karamanoukian, R.; Papazian, N. Burn injury: Review of pathophysiology and therapeutic modalities in major burns. *Ann. Burn. Fire Disasters* **2017**, *30*, 95–102.
21. Scuderi, N.; Dessy, L.A.; Buccheri, E.M.; Marchetti, F.; Mazzocchi, M.; Chiummariello, S.; Klinger, F.; Onesti, M.G.; Klinger, M.; Alfano, C. Phase 2 cross-over multicenter trial on the efficacy and safety of topical cyanoacrylates compared with topical silicone gel in the prevention of pathologic scars. *Aesthetic Plast. Surg.* **2011**, *35*, 373–381. [CrossRef] [PubMed]
22. Illario, M. Good practices for a "Decade for Active and Healthy Ageing. *Transl. Med. UniSa* **2020**, *23*, 16. [CrossRef]
23. Bulla, A.; Bolletta, A.; Fiorot, L.; Maffei, M.; Bandiera, P.; Casoli, V.; Montella, A.; Campus, G.V. Posterior tibial perforators relationship with superficial nerves and veins: A cadaver study. *Microsurgery* **2019**, *39*, 241–246. [CrossRef] [PubMed]
24. Mansueto, G.; De Simone, M.; Ciamarra, P.; Capasso, E.; Feola, A.; Campobasso, C.P. Infections Are a Very Dangerous Affair: Enterobiasis and Death. *Healthcare* **2021**, *9*, 1641. [CrossRef] [PubMed]
25. Dovedytis, M.; Liu, Z.J.; Bartlett, S. Hyaluronic acid and its biomedical applications: A review. *Eng. Regen.* **2020**, *1*, 102–113. [CrossRef]
26. Rosen, J.; Landriscina, A.; Kutner, A.; Adler, B.L.; Krausz, A.E.; Nosanchuk, J.D.; Friedman, A.J. Silver sulfadiazine retards wound healing in mice via alterations in cytokine expression. *J. Investig. Dermatol.* **2015**, *135*, 1459–1462. [CrossRef]
27. Oaks, R.J.; Cindass, R. Silver Sulfadiazine. In *StatPearls*; StatPearls Publishing: Treasure Island, FL, USA, 2022.
28. Tito, A.; Minale, M.; Riccio, S.; Grieco, F.; Colucci, M.G.; Apone, F. A *Triticum vulgare* Extract Exhibits Regenerating Activity During the Wound Healing Process. *Clin. Cosmet. Investig. Dermatol.* **2020**, *13*, 21–30. [CrossRef]
29. Fiore, L.; Scapagnini, U.; Riccio, R.; Canonico, P.L. Differential activities of Triticum vulgare extract and its fractions in mouse fibroblasts. *Acta Ther.* **1993**, *19*, 151–162.
30. Morretta, E.; D'Agostino, A.; Cassese, E.; Maglione, B.; Petrella, A.; Schiraldi, C.; Monti, M.C. Label-Free Quantitative Proteomics to Explore the Action Mechanism of the Pharmaceutical-Grade *Triticum vulgare* Extract in Speeding Up Keratinocyte Healing. *Molecules* **2022**, *27*, 1108. [CrossRef]
31. Kaehn, K. Polihexanide: A safe and highly effective biocide. *Skin Pharmacol. Physiol.* **2010**, *23*, 7–16. [CrossRef]
32. Lo Torto, F.L.; Losco, L.; Bernardini, N.; Greco, M.; Scuderi, G.; Ribuffo, D. Surgical Treatment with Locoregional Flaps for the Eyelid: A Review. *BioMed Res. Int.* **2017**, *2017*, 6742537. [CrossRef] [PubMed]
33. Losco, L.; Aksoyler, D.; Chen, S.H.; Bolletta, A.; Velazquez-Mujica, J.; Di Taranto, G.; Lo Torto, F.; Marcasciano, M.; Cigna, E.; Chen, H.C. Pharyngoesophageal reconstruction with free jejunum or radial forearm flap as diversionary conduit: Functional outcomes of patients with persistent dysphagia and aspiration. *Microsurgery* **2020**, *40*, 630–638. [CrossRef] [PubMed]
34. Gazzabin, L.; Serantoni, S.; Palumbo, F.P.; Giordan, N. Hyaluronic acid and metallic silver treatment of chronic wounds: Healing rate and bacterial load control. *J. Wound Care* **2019**, *28*, 482–490. [CrossRef] [PubMed]
35. Kaciulyte, J.; Garutti, L.; Spadoni, D.; Velazquez-Mujica, J.; Losco, L.; Ciudad, P.; Marcasciano, M.; Lo Torto, F.; Casella, D.; Ribuffo, D.; et al. Genital Lymphedema and How to Deal with It: Pearls and Pitfalls from over 38 Years of Experience with Unusual Lymphatic System Impairment. *Medicina* **2021**, *57*, 1175. [CrossRef] [PubMed]
36. Maruccia, M.; Onesti, M.G.; Sorvillo, V.; Albano, A.; Dessy, L.A.; Carlesimo, B.; Tarallo, M.; Marcasciano, M.; Giudice, G.; Cigna, E.; et al. An Alternative Treatment Strategy for Complicated Chronic Wounds: Negative Pressure Therapy over Mesh Skin Graft. *BioMed Res. Int.* **2017**, *2017*, 8395219. [CrossRef] [PubMed]
37. Chiummariello, S.; Del Torto, G.; Iera, M.; Arleo, S.; Alfano, C. Negative pressure dressing in split-thickness skin grafts: Experience with an alternative method. *Wounds* **2013**, *25*, 324–327.
38. Costagliola, M.; Agrosi, M. Second-degree burns: A comparative, multicenter, randomized trial of hyaluronic acid plus silver sulfadiazine vs. silver sulfadiazine alone. *Curr. Med. Res. Opin.* **2005**, *21*, 1235–1240. [CrossRef]
39. Voigt, J.; Driver, V.R. Hyaluronic acid derivatives and their healing effect on burns, epithelial surgical wounds, and chronic wounds: A systematic review and meta-analysis of randomized controlled trials. *Wound Repair Regen.* **2012**, *20*, 317–331. [CrossRef]
40. Martini, P.; Mazzatenta, C.; Saponati, G. Efficacy and tolerability of fitostimoline in two different forms (soaked gauzes and cream) and citrizan gel in the topical treatment of second-degree superficial cutaneous burns. *Dermatol. Res. Pract.* **2011**, *2011*, 978291. [CrossRef]
41. Clark, R.A. Fibrin and wound healing. *Ann. N. Y. Acad. Sci.* **2001**, *936*, 355–367. [CrossRef]
42. Amrani, D.L.; Diorio, J.P.; Delmotte, Y. Wound healing. Role of commercial fibrin sealants. *Ann. N. Y. Acad. Sci.* **2001**, *936*, 566–579. [CrossRef] [PubMed]

43. Van Hinsbergh, V.W.; Collen, A.; Koolwijk, P. Role of fibrin matrix in angiogenesis. *Ann. N. Y. Acad. Sci.* **2001**, *936*, 426–437. [CrossRef]
44. Yaftali, N.A.; Weber, K. Corticosteroids and Hyaluronic Acid Injections. *Clin. Sports Med.* **2019**, *38*, 1–15. [CrossRef] [PubMed]
45. Parihar, A.; Parihar, M.S.; Milner, S.; Bhat, S. Oxidative stress and anti-oxidative mobilization in burn injury. *Burns* **2008**, *34*, 6–17. [CrossRef]
46. Petrey, A.C.; De La Motte, C.A. Hyaluronan, a crucial regulator of inflammation. *Front. Immunol.* **2014**, *5*, 101. [CrossRef]
47. Caruso, A.; Cutuli, V.M.; De Bernardis, E.; Amico-Roxas, M. Protective action of epidermal growth factor and a fraction from Triticum vulgare extract in mouse tail necrosis. *Life Sci.* **1997**, *60*, PL175–PL180. [CrossRef]
48. D'Agostino, A.; Pirozzi, A.V.A.; Finamore, R.; Grieco, F.; Minale, M.; Schiraldi, C. Molecular Mechanisms at the Basis of Pharmaceutical Grade Triticum vulgare Extract Efficacy in Prompting Keratinocytes Healing. *Molecules* **2020**, *25*, 431. [CrossRef] [PubMed]
49. Cantisani, C.; Paolino, G.; Scarnò, M.; Didona, D.; Tallarico, M.; Moliterni, E.; Losco, L.; Cantoresi, F.; Mercuri, S.R.; Bottoniτ, U.; et al. Sequential methyl-aminolevulinate daylight photodynamic therapy and diclofenac plus hyaluronic acid gel treatment for multiple actinic keratosis evaluation. *Dermatol. Ther.* **2018**, *31*, e12710. [CrossRef]
50. Tiwari, V.K. Burn wound: How it differs from other wounds? *Indian J. Plast. Surg.* **2012**, *45*, 364–373. [CrossRef]
51. Jeschke, M.G.; Van Baar, M.E.; Choudhry, M.A.; Chung, K.K.; Gibran, N.S.; Logsetty, S. Burn injury. *Nat. Rev. Dis. Primers* **2020**, *6*, 11. [CrossRef]

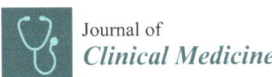

Article

Modified Mini-Keystone Flaps for Coverage of Tiny Volar Pulp Defects of the Fingertips in Cases with Missing Amputation Skin Stumps: A Retrospective Study

Byung Woo Yoo [†], Seungyoon Oh [†], Junekyu Kim, Kap Sung Oh, Hyun Woo Shin [†] and Kyu Nam Kim *

Department of Plastic and Reconstructive Surgery, Kangbuk Samsung Hospital,
Sungkyunkwan University School of Medicine, 29, Saemunan-ro, Jongno-gu, Seoul 03181, Korea;
dbansdj@naver.com (B.W.Y.); yoona1507@gmail.com (S.O.); kokoro72@naver.com (J.K.);
kapsung.oh@samsung.com (K.S.O.); mdshin7@naver.com (H.W.S.)
* Correspondence: manabear77@naver.com; Tel.: +82-10-6485-0584
† These authors contributed equally to this work.

Abstract: This study aimed to demonstrate the expanding versatility of keystone flap reconstruction in fingertips. Fifteen patients who underwent the modified mini-keystone flap reconstruction for tiny volar pulp defects of the fingertip between September 2020 and February 2021 were included in this study (average age: 43.4 ± 13.52 years, range: 19–61 years). Patient data were retrospectively collected from their medical records. The two-point discrimination test was used to evaluate the degree of sensory recovery. All defects were successfully covered with the modified mini-keystone flap. The defect sizes ranged from 0.5 cm × 1 cm to 1.2 cm × 2.0 cm, and the flap sizes ranged from 0.7 cm × 1.5 cm to 1.5 cm × 3.0 cm. Although one patient showed a small distal margin maceration, all flaps survived fully. The overall outcomes were favorable at the mean follow-up period of 5.73 ± 0.79 months. We suggest that the modified mini-keystone flap technique is a promising alternative modality for covering tiny volar pulp defects of the fingertip, with few complications and favorable outcomes.

Keywords: fingertip defect; tiny defect; volar pulp defect; keystone flap; flap coverage

1. Introduction

Fingertip defects are common injuries of the upper extremities because the fingertip is the most peripheral part of the body. However, treatment of these injuries is challenging because of the prominent role of the fingertips in an individual's activities [1]. In particular, tiny volar pulp defects of the fingertips are a common problem in daily life. Tiny defects can be defined as very small wounds for which primary closure is difficult to achieve due to the loss of some skin and soft tissues and reduction in elasticity in their location. These defects are often caused by trauma, such as cuts with a knife, saw, or sharp edge. In cases with an existing amputation skin stump, a skin graft using the stump is the best option for coverage. However, when amputation skin stumps are unavailable, several methods, such as conservative dressing, skin grafts from other donor sites, and local flaps, can be used. Each of these techniques have both advantages and disadvantages. In the absence of an ideal method, a particular defect can be managed using various options to yield similar results [2,3]. Generally, superficial defects can be covered with skin grafts, and flap techniques are useful to cover deep defects with exposure of the underlying structures [3]. Surgeons usually choose an appropriate reconstructive method on a case-by-case basis according to the location and size of each defect [4]. Although various flap techniques have been devised to cover fingertip defects, new or modified techniques can yield favorable or better outcomes compared with previous methods. Herein, we present a retrospective review of our clinical experience with tiny volar pulp defect coverage using a modified mini-keystone flap (m-KF), that is, a combination of omega variation (OV) closure and Sydney Melanoma Unit Modification (SMUM). Through this study, we demonstrate the expanding versatility of KF reconstruction in fingertips.

2. Materials and Methods

This study was approved by the Institutional Review Board of our hospital. All research procedures in this study were performed in accordance with the guidelines proposed in the 1975 Declaration of Helsinki. All the patients in this study provided written consent to publish their information and images in an online open access publication before undergoing the procedures and operations.

In this study, we included patients who underwent modified m-KF reconstruction for tiny volar pulp defects of the fingertip between September 2020 and February 2021. Patients who underwent fingertip defect reconstruction using other methods, such as skin grafts and other flaps, were excluded. Patients' data from medical records and clinical photographs were retrospectively reviewed to obtain information regarding defect causes, defect locations, defect sizes, flap sizes, flap survival, complications, two-point discrimination test (2-PDT) results, and the findings of follow-up assessments for each patient. We routinely obtained 2-PDT measurements to evaluate the degree of sensory recovery at the final postoperative follow-up of each patient.

2.1. Surgical Techniques

After debridement of the lesion of the fingertip, the final defect was identified, and modified m-KF reconstruction was performed. This flap was named m-KF because it was much smaller than the ubiquitous KF. We used OV closure [5] and SMUM [6] KF in all cases. The OV KF is a modification of the conventional KF in which the original defect is closed in a fish-mouth fashion through additional rotational movement [4,5,7]. The SMUM KF entails maintaining a skin bridge along the greater arch of the KF [4,6,7]. The modified m-KF was designed to be slightly larger than the defect at the side of sufficient tissue laxity. A skin incision was made along the flap with the remaining skin bridge, and dissection progressed to the subcutaneous tissues. The flap margin was minimally undermined to achieve OV closure. Fastidious hemostasis was achieved, and flap inset was performed in the following sequence: a three-point area (tip of a fish-mouth closure) of the OV was sutured first, both ends of the V-Y closure were sutured next, and the donor side (greater arc) of the m-KF was sutured at the end. A simple dressing with foam material was applied at the end of the operation. Figure 1 presents the schematic diagrams of the modified m-KF reconstruction for tiny volar pulp defects of the fingertip.

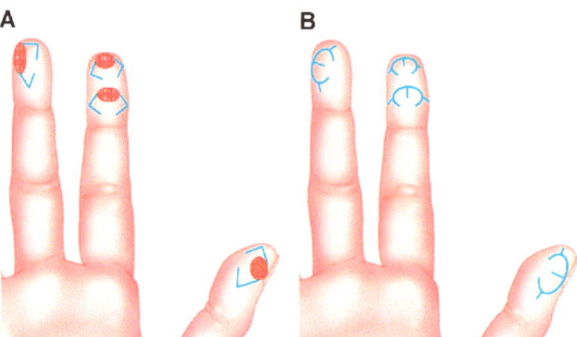

Figure 1. Schematic diagrams of modified mini-keystone flap (m-KF) reconstruction for tiny volar defects of the fingertip. (**A**) Various tiny volar defects of the fingertips (red-colored ovals) and designs of the modified m-KFs (blue-colored lines). (**B**) Final appearance after coverage of the modified m-KFs (blue-colored lines).

2.2. Evaluation of Postoperative Functional Outcomes

We recorded the degree of sensory recovery at the final postoperative follow-up examination by using the Touch Test® 2-Point Discriminator (North Coast Medical Inc., Morgan Hill, CA, USA) to measure static and dynamic two-point discrimination. All tests were performed and recorded for the flap coverage area of the affected fingertip and the equivalent area of the contralateral normal fingertip by our senior author. For the static two-point discrimination test (2-PDT), values of <6 mm, 6–10 mm, and >11 mm indicated good, fair, and poor discrimination, respectively [8–10]. For the dynamic 2-PDT, values of <4 mm, 4–7 mm, and >8 mm indicated good, fair, and poor discrimination, respectively [8–10]. Figure 2 shows the two-point discriminator and the 2-PDT setup used in this study.

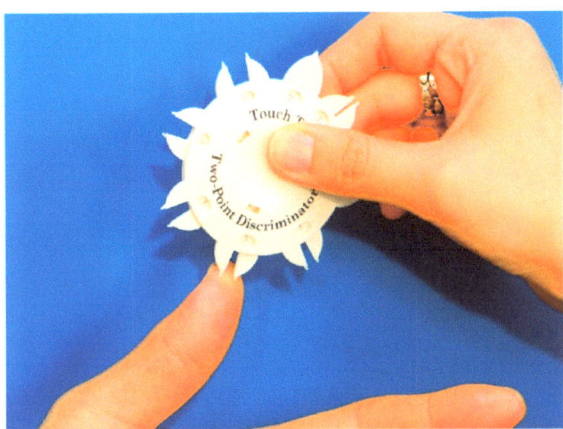

Figure 2. The two-point discrimination test (2-PDT). To perform the 2-PDT, the evaluator touches the patient's fingertip with the two-point discriminator device, randomly alternating between one and two points. The patient is asked to report whether one or two points were felt.

2.3. Statistical Analysis

We used GraphPad Prism version 8.4.3 (GraphPad Software Inc., San Diego, CA, USA) software for all statistical analyses. Continuous variables were expressed as mean ± standard deviation (SD). We used Student's t-test for continuous variables to compare the differences between 2-PDT at the affected fingertip and that at the contralateral normal fingertip. The significance level was set at $p < 0.05$.

3. Results

The patients' clinical data are summarized in Table 1. A total of 15 patients (10 male and 5 female patients) aged 19–61 years (average age, 43.4 ± 13.52 years) were included in this study. The defects were caused by traumatic injury in all cases. All defects corresponded to the aforementioned definition of a tiny full-thickness defect with no bone exposure. The sizes of the defects ranged from 0.5 cm × 1.0 cm to 1.2 cm × 2.0 cm. Successful coverage of all defects was achieved by using m-KF combined with OV and SMUM. The flap sizes ranged from 0.7 cm × 1.5 cm to 1.5 cm × 3.0 cm. All flaps survived without any flap-related complications, such as venous congestion and arterial insufficiency. One patient had small-sized macerations of the distal margin; however, this was resolved with conservative treatment and required no further surgical management. All other patients were completely healed without any wound complications at 2-week postoperative follow-up. At the average follow-up period of 5.73 ± 0.79 months (range, 5–7 months), the mean static 2-PDT value at the affected and the contralateral normal fingertips were 4.00 ± 1.13 mm and 3.60 ± 0.63 mm, respectively ($p = 0.243$). The mean dynamic 2-PDT value at the affected and contralateral normal fingertips were 3.27 ± 1.03 mm and 2.87 ± 0.64 mm, respectively

($p = 0.213$). All 2-PDT values were above fair, and all patients were adequately satisfied with their final outcomes. Table 2 summarizes the 2-PDT data. In the following section (Case Presentations), we describe some representative cases to elucidate our m-KF reconstruction method for tiny volar pulp defects in fingertips.

Table 1. Patients' data.

Case	Age/Sex	Cause of the Defect	Defect Location	Defect Size (cm^2)	Flap Size (cm^2)	Flap Survival	Complications	Static 2-PDT (Affected Fingertip/Contralateral Normal Fingertip, mm)	Dynamic 2-PDT (Affected Fingertip/Contralateral Normal Fingertip, mm)	Follow-Up Period (Months)
1	F/27	Trauma caused by cutter knife	Rt. volar pulp of the thumb	0.7 × 1.0	0.9 × 2.0	Fully survived	None	3/3	2/2	7
2	F/59	Trauma caused by kitchen knife	Lt. volar pulp of the fifth finger	0.5 × 1.0	0.7 × 1.5	Fully survived	None	4/4	3/3	6
3	M/61	Trauma caused by cutter knife	Rt. volar pulp of the thumb	1.0 × 1.5	1.5 × 3.0	Fully survived	Distal margin maceration	6/4	5/3	5
4	M/34	Trauma caused by cutter knife	Lt. volar pulp of the fourth finger	0.7 × 0.9	0.9 × 1.6	Fully survived	None	3/3	2/2	7
5	M/47	Trauma caused by cutter knife	Rt. volar pulp of the second finger	0.6 × 1.0	0.8 × 1.5	Fully survived	None	2/2	2/2	6
6	M/36	Trauma caused by cutter knife	Lt. volar pulp of the fifth finger	0.6 × 1.5	0.8 × 2.5	Fully survived	None	4/4	3/3	6
7	M/19	Trauma caused by cutter knife	Rt. volar pulp of the thumb	0.8 × 1.1	1.0 × 2.3	Fully survived	None	3/3	2/2	7
8	M/41	Trauma caused by kitchen knife	Lt. volar pulp of the second finger	0.6 × 1.0	0.8 × 2.0	Fully survived	None	4/4	3/3	6
9	M/58	Trauma caused by cutter knife	Rt. volar pulp of the second finger	0.9 × 1.5	1.3 × 2.5	Fully survived	None	4/4	4/4	5

Table 1. Cont.

Case	Age/Sex	Cause of the Defect	Defect Location	Defect Size (cm^2)	Flap Size (cm^2)	Flap Survival	Complications	Static 2-PDT (Affected Fingertip/Contralateral Normal Fingertip, mm)	Dynamic 2-PDT (Affected Fingertip/Contralateral Normal Fingertip, mm)	Follow-Up Period (Months)
10	M/56	Trauma caused by cutter knife	Lt. volar pulp of the second finger	0.6 × 1.2	0.9 × 1.6	Fully survived	None	5/4	4/3	5
11	M/30	Trauma caused by kitchen knife	Lt. volar pulp of the thumb	1.2 × 2.0	1.5 × 3.0	Fully survived	None	6/4	5/3	5
12	M/31	Trauma caused by kitchen knife	Lt. volar pulp of the second finger	0.7 × 1.2	1.0 × 2.2	Fully survived	None	3/3	3/3	5
13	F/42	Trauma caused by cutter knife	Rt. volar pulp of the fifth finger	0.6 × 1.1	0.8 × 1.7	Fully survived	None	4/4	4/4	5
14	F/56	Trauma caused by kitchen knife	Rt. volar pulp of the fourth finger	0.7 × 1.3	1.1 × 1.8	Fully survived	None	4/4	3/3	5
15	F/54	Trauma caused by kitchen knife	Lt. volar pulp of the second finger	0.8 × 1.0	1.2 × 2.0	Fully survived	None	5/4	4/3	6

F, female; M, male; Rt., right; Lt., left; 2-PDT, two-point discrimination test.

Table 2. Summary of the two-point discrimination test data.

	Static 2-PDT (Affected Fingertip)	Static 2-PDT (Contralateral Normal Fingertip)	Dynamic 2-PDT (Affected Fingertip)	Dynamic 2-PDT (Contralateral Normal Fingertip)
Good (Static 2-PDT, <6 mm; dynamic 2-PDT, <4 mm)	13	15	8	13
Fair (Static 2-PDT, 6~10 mm; dynamic 2-PDT, 4~7 mm)	2	0	7	2
Poor (Static 2-PDT, >10 mm; dynamic 2-PDT, >7 mm)	0	0	0	0
Mean ± SD (mm)	4.00 ± 1.13	3.60 ± 0.63	3.27 ± 1.03	2.87 ± 0.64
Student's t-test	$p = 0.243$		$p = 0.213$	

2-PDT, two-point discrimination test; SD, standard deviation.

3.1. Case Presentations

3.1.1. Case 5

A 47-year-old man sustained a right second fingertip injury while using a cutter knife. The patient's amputation skin stump was not available. Under a digital nerve block, we performed debridement and identified a 0.6 cm × 1.0 cm sized tiny volar pulp defect (Figure 3). We covered the defect with a modified m-KF (0.8 cm × 1.5 cm) from the proximal side of the defect. Flap insertion and donor-site closure with minimal tension were achieved. The flap fully survived without any postoperative complications. At the 6-month follow-up, the static 2-PDT value was 2 mm in the affected fingertip and 2 mm in the contralateral normal fingertip, and the dynamic 2-PDT value was 2 mm in the affected fingertip and 2 mm in the contralateral normal fingertip. The patient was satisfied with the final outcome.

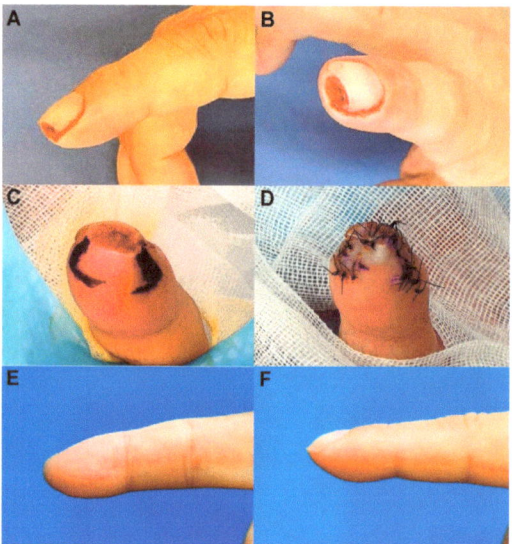

Figure 3. Clinical photographs of a 47-year-old man who sustained a right second fingertip injury while using a cutter knife. (**A,B**) A tiny volar pulp defect of the right second fingertip (0.6 cm × 1 cm). (**C**) Design of a modified mini-keystone flap (m-KF) (0.8 cm × 1.5 cm). (**D**) Successful coverage of the defect with the modified m-KF. (**E,F**) Postoperative photographs obtained at the 6-month follow-up.

3.1.2. Case 6

A 36-year-old man sustained a left fifth fingertip injury while using a cutter knife. The patient's amputation skin stump was unavailable. Under a digital nerve block, we performed debridement and identified a 0.6 cm × 1.5 cm sized tiny volar pulp defect (Figure 4). The defect was covered with a modified m-KF (0.8 cm × 2.5 cm) from the proximal side of the defect. Flap insertion and donor-site closure with minimal tension were achieved. The flap survived without any postoperative complications. At the 6-month follow-up, the static 2-PDT value was 4 mm in both the affected fingertip and the contralateral normal fingertip, while the dynamic 2-PDT value was 3 mm in both the affected and contralateral normal fingertips. The patient was satisfied with the final outcome.

3.1.3. Case 11

A 30-year-old man sustained a left thumb fingertip injury while using a kitchen knife. The patient's amputation skin stump was unavailable. Under a digital nerve block, we performed debridement and identified a 1.2 cm × 2.0 cm sized tiny volar pulp defect (Figure 5). We covered the defect using a modified m-KF (1.5 cm × 3.0 cm) from the proximal side of the defect. Flap insertion and donor-site closure with minimal tension were achieved. The flap survived without any postoperative complications. At the 5-month follow-up, the static 2-PDT value was 6 mm in the affected fingertip and 4 mm in the contralateral normal fingertip, and the dynamic 2-PDT value was 5 mm in the affected fingertip and 3 mm in the contralateral normal fingertip. The patient was satisfied with the final outcome.

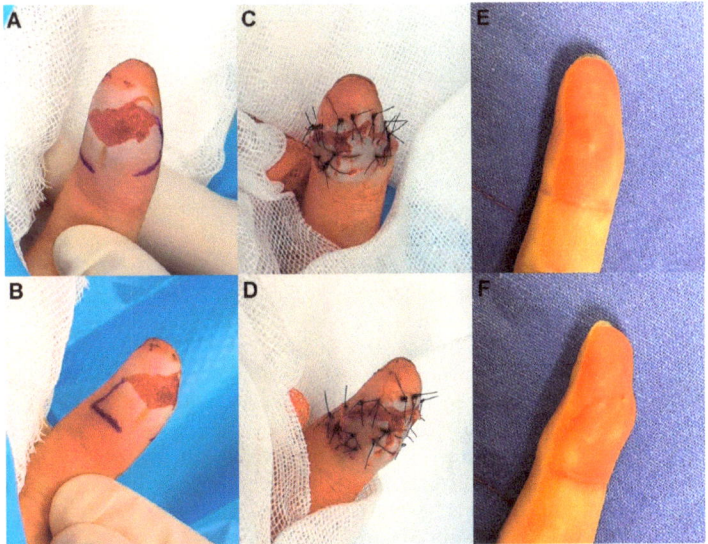

Figure 4. Clinical photographs of a 36-year-old man who sustained a left fifth fingertip injury caused by a cutter knife. (**A,B**) A tiny volar pulp defect of the right second fingertip (0.6 cm × 1.5 cm), and design of a modified mini-keystone flap (m-KF) (0.8 × 2.5 cm). (**C,D**) Successful coverage of the defect with the modified m-KF. (**E,F**) Postoperative photographs obtained at the 6-month follow-up.

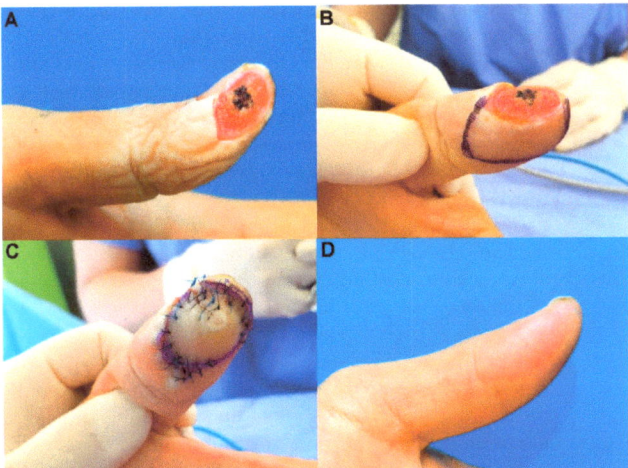

Figure 5. Clinical photographs of a 30-year-old man who sustained a left thumb fingertip injury while using a kitchen knife. (**A**) A tiny volar pulp defect of the left thumb fingertip (1.2 cm × 2.0 cm). (**B**) Design of a modified mini-keystone flap (m-KF) (1.5 cm × 3.0 cm). (**C**) Successful coverage of the defect with the modified m-KF. (**D**) Postoperative photographs obtained at the 5-month follow-up.

4. Discussion

This retrospective study reports our successful experience with modified m-KF reconstruction for tiny volar pulp defects of the fingertips. As mentioned earlier, a wide variety of reconstructive options have been developed for fingertip defects, with scarce evidence supporting one method over the other [2]. Therefore, the ideal treatment for different types of fingertip injuries remains debatable [1,2,11,12]. Generally, the fundamental reconstructive principles include replacing like-with-like tissues, minimizing donor-site morbidity, and recovering normal functional properties. Considering these objectives, free flaps are suitable for large fingertip reconstruction, whereas local flaps can be the best choice for small-to-moderate-sized defect coverage of the fingertip [1,2,11]. A variety of local flaps can be used to cover fingertip defects [1,2,11]. V-Y advancement flaps, rotation flaps, transposition flaps, and bilobed flaps can be used to cover small-sized fingertip defects [1,2,11,13]. However, homo-digital and hetero-digital island flaps, cross-finger flaps, and dorsal metacarpal artery perforator flaps are required to cover moderate-sized defects in the fingers [2,14,15].

KF, devised by Behan in 2003, is one of the most meaningful innovations in the field of reconstructive surgery over the last 20 years [3,4,7,16]. KF is characterized by its simple and defect-adaptive design, with a curvilinear-shaped trapezoidal design consisting of two conjoined V-Y flaps moving in the horizontal direction on the longitudinal flap axis [3,4,7,16]. A large number of studies have shown that KF reconstruction can cover various anatomical defects in the human body, including the head, neck, trunk, and extremities [4,7,16–18]. In contrast, only a few reports have described KF finger reconstruction [19,20]. Although no previous article has described KF fingertip reconstruction, a literature review using PubMed and Google Scholar with search terms including "keystone flap" AND "finger" identified two articles describing KF finger reconstruction, which were case reports [19,20]. To the best of our knowledge, our study presents the first case series of KF reconstruction for fingertip defects.

The original classification of KF by Behan covered four subtypes: type I (skin incision only), type II (A, division of the deep fascia along the outer curvilinear line; B, division of the deep fascia and skin graft to the secondary defect), type III (opposing keystone flaps designed to create a double-keystone flap), and type IV (keystone flap with undermining of up to 50% of the flap subfascially) [16]. In addition to these original subtypes, two representative modifications have been devised: the OV KF and the SMUM KF [4–7]. As mentioned earlier, we used a combination of OV and SMUM KFs in all cases of the present study. The OV KF can provide further flap movement via additional rotational movement as mentioned above, and, consequently, it can reduce tension as well as avoid sacrifice of healthy tissues during wound closure [4,5,7]. SMUM KF can allow additional vascularity, preserve the subdermal lymphatics, and provide structural stabilization of the flap through the skin bridge [4,6,7]. When small-sized flaps for covering tiny defects are applied as m-KFs, these two modifications are very helpful in acquiring sufficient flap movement and maintaining hemodynamic flap stability while performing minimal undermining of the flap. Through the combination of these two modifications, we achieved complete flap survival with no significant postoperative complications in all of our cases.

In tiny volar pulp defects of the fingertip, skin grafts using the amputation skin stump are generally used as a simple and optimal option; however, this option is frequently not available due to the absence of the skin stump or because of contaminated amputation [1]. In such cases, three treatment methods, namely, secondary intention with conservative dressing, skin graft from another donor site, and local flaps, can be considered. Secondary intention with conservative dressing, such as occlusive or semi-occlusive dressing, may actually represent the simplest solution for any small and superficial fingertip defects that do not involve the bone. However, it is usually a time-consuming treatment method and is often compromised by delayed wound healing due to an underlying disease or concurrent wound infection. Furthermore, patients may complain of persistent pain until epithelialization progresses to some extent. Through fingertip defect coverage with skin graft and local flap, surgeons can perform more time-saving treatment methods and achieve reliable wound healing for patients. Skin grafts are commonly used to cover defects of various sizes without exposure of vital structures in reconstructive surgery [3,7]. However, they have some limitations, including vulnerability to mechanical forces, decreased sensation, color and texture mismatch, and donor-site morbidity [3,7]. Reconstruction with the local flap technique is superior to other options because it allows reconstruction of the volar pulp in the fingertip with a tissue showing similar features [1,21]. The volar pulp skin of the fingertip comes under a lot of weight during hand function because of its specialized sensation and grasp abilities [1]. Thus, the ideal reconstruction outcomes of the volar pulp area can be achieved by coverage with local tissues that have similar skin durability while preserving sensation [1,21]. In the present study, our modified m-KF technique for covering tiny volar defects of the fingertip yielded favorable outcomes in all cases. In particular, the functional outcomes of our study were remarkable in terms of sensation recovery. The mean values of both the static and dynamic 2-PDT at the affected fingertip did not show a significant difference from the corresponding values at the contralateral normal fingertip in the present study ($p = 0.243$ and $p = 0.213$) (Figure 6). Furthermore, all 2-PDT values were more than fair in all cases. On the basis of these results, we inferred that the modified m-KF technique can provide outstanding sensation recovery in tiny volar pulp reconstruction.

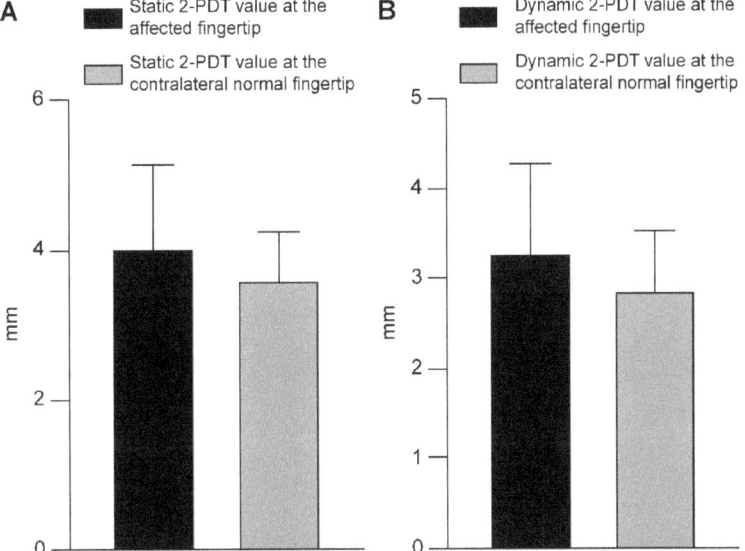

Figure 6. Comparison of mean differences between continuous variables in the two-point discrimination test (2-PDT) data. (**A**) Static 2-PDT. (**B**) Dynamic 2-PDT.

Because fingers perform various movements and lack sufficient surrounding tissues, securing minimal wound tension when covering finger defects is very important [19]. An attempt to close the defect under tension can result in a high risk of wound-related complications [19]. Although the volar pulp area of the fingertip has a relatively consistent amount of tissue compared with that of other finger regions, closing the wound without tension is still difficult, and wound closure with minimal tension is obviously essential. Recruitment and rearrangement of tissue laxity is a crucial biomechanical property of KF reconstruction, which results from the use of two conjoined V-Y advancement flaps at each end of the KF by redistributing the wound tension perpendicular to the line of advancement [4,7,18]. This redistribution of the wound tension results in a tension-reducing effect of KF in wound closure [4,7,18]. In the present study, we considered that the modified m-KF technique also allowed the wound to be closed with minimal tension when covering tiny volar defects despite the limited amount of extra tissue in the fingertip. Thus, there were no significant wound problems requiring surgical intervention or revision in our cases. All surgical procedures and postoperative care in this study were performed in the outpatient clinic, indicating that the modified m-KF technique is simple and convenient.

Despite the successful outcomes, our study had several limitations. This study included a very small number of cases, was a nonrandomized retrospective study, and had no comparison group. Therefore, selection bias and confounding factors were inevitably encountered, which affected the study outcomes. A well-designed prospective large-scale study with other comparison groups is required to confirm the favorable and consistent outcomes of our study. Meanwhile, with regard to the choice of reconstructive surgery, our modified m-KF is not an optimal method, although it can be a reliable alternative for fingertip defects. Reconstructive surgeons do not have to adhere to the use of the modified m-KF for the reconstruction of tiny fingertip defects in all cases. Finally, any scar at the volar pulp of the fingertip can be painful and irritating for patients. Limited aesthetic results, such as change in fingertip contour, can occur due to surgical reconstructions; therefore, surgical procedures such as our modified m-KF should be performed with caution. As mentioned earlier, we designed the flap at the side of sufficient tissue laxity (Figure 1). The abovementioned tension-reducing effect of the modified m-KF can allow wound closure with minimal tension, possibly helping in minimizing scar formation in the volar pulp area. Despite these limitations, our study findings are significant because this study is the first consecutive case series that describes fingertip defect reconstruction using KF conducted by a single surgeon (the corresponding author of this study) and demonstrates the expanding versatility of KF in reconstructive surgery.

5. Conclusions

Based on the successful outcomes reported in this study, we believe that the modified m-KF technique can be a good alternative to other reconstructive modalities for covering tiny volar pulp defects of the fingertip in terms of assurance of reliable outcomes (outstanding sensation recovery) and fulfillment of ideal reconstruction (replacement of like-with-like tissue). Furthermore, we plan to apply KF reconstruction to other finger and hand regions to enhance and expand the usefulness of the KF technique based on our study findings.

Author Contributions: Conceptualization, K.N.K.; methodology, K.N.K. and H.W.S.; data curation, B.W.Y. and S.O.; formal analysis, K.N.K., H.W.S. and B.W.Y.; writing—original draft preparation, B.W.Y. and S.O.; supervision, J.K. and K.S.O.; writing—review and editing, K.N.K. and H.W.S. All authors have read and agreed to the published version of the manuscript.

Funding: This research received no external funding.

Institutional Review Board Statement: The study was conducted in accordance with the Declaration of Helsinki, and approved by the Institutional Review Board (or Ethics Committee) of Kangbuk Samsung Hospital (approval number: 2021-04-039-001; date of approval: 7 May 2021).

Informed Consent Statement: Written informed consent was obtained from all subjects involved in the study. Written informed consent has also been obtained from the patients to publish this paper.

Data Availability Statement: The data presented in this study are available on request from the corresponding author. The data are not publicly available due to privacy restrictions.

Acknowledgments: We would like to thank Ji Hyun Chang from Seoul National University Hospital for performing the statistical analysis of this study.

Conflicts of Interest: The authors declare no conflict of interest.

References

1. Ozturk, M.B.; Barutca, S.A.; Aksan, T.; Atik, B. Pulp rotation flap for lateral oblique fingertip defects. *Ann. Plast. Surg.* **2016**, *77*, 529–534. [CrossRef] [PubMed]
2. Das De, S.; Sebastin, S.J. Soft tissue coverage of the digits and hand. *Hand Clin.* **2020**, *36*, 97–105. [CrossRef] [PubMed]

3. Yoon, C.S.; Kim, S.I.; Kim, H.; Kim, K.N. Keystone-designed perforator island flaps for the coverage of traumatic pretibial defects in patients with comorbidities. *Int. J. Low. Extrem. Wounds* **2017**, *16*, 302–309. [CrossRef] [PubMed]
4. Lim, S.Y.; Yoon, C.S.; Lee, H.G.; Kim, K.N. Keystone design perforator island flap in facial defect reconstruction. *World J. Clin. Cases* **2020**, *8*, 1832–1847. [CrossRef] [PubMed]
5. Behan, F.C.; Rozen, W.M.; Lo, C.H.; Findlay, M. The omega—Ω—variant designs (types A and B) of the keystone perforator island flap. *ANZ J. Surg.* **2011**, *81*, 650–652. [CrossRef] [PubMed]
6. Moncrieff, M.D.; Bowen, F.; Thompson, J.F.; Saw, R.P.; Shannon, K.F.; Spillane, A.J.; Quinn, M.J.; Stretch, J.R. Keystone flap reconstruction of primary melanoma excision defects of the leg –the end of the skin graft? *Ann. Surg. Oncol.* **2008**, *15*, 2867–2873. [CrossRef]
7. Lee, H.G.; Lim, S.Y.; Kim, Y.K.; Yoon, C.S.; Kim, K.N. Keystone design perforator island flaps for coverage of non-oncological periarticular defects surrounded by the zone of injury. *J. Int. Med. Res.* **2020**, *48*, 0300060520930152. [CrossRef]
8. Lundborg, G.; Rosén, B. The two-point discrimination test–time for a re-appraisal? *J. Hand Surg. Br.* **2004**, *29*, 418–422. [CrossRef]
9. Silva, P.G.; Jones, A.; Araujo, P.M.; Natour, J. Assessment of light touch sensation in the hands of systemic sclerosis patients. *Clinics* **2014**, *69*, 585–588. [CrossRef]
10. Weber, R.A.; Breidenbach, W.C.; Brown, R.E.; Jabaley, M.E.; Mass, D.P. A randomized prospective study of polyglycolic acid conduits for digital nerve reconstruction in humans. *Plast. Reconstr. Surg.* **2000**, *106*, 1036–1045, discussion 1046. [CrossRef]
11. Kawaiah, A.; Thakur, M.; Garg, S.; Kawasmi, S.H.; Hassan, A. Fingertip injuries and amputations: A review of the literature. *Cureus* **2020**, *12*, e8291. [CrossRef] [PubMed]
12. Moon, S.H.; Jung, S.N.; Kim, H.J.; Kwon, H.; Sohn, W.I.; Yoo, G.; Im, K.S. Treatment of posttraumatic fingertip pain using a great toe pulp graft. *Ann. Plast. Surg.* **2011**, *67*, 25–29. [CrossRef] [PubMed]
13. Gharb, B.B.; Rampazzo, A.; Armijo, B.S.; Eshraghi, Y.; Totonchi, A.S.; Teo, T.C.; Salgado, C.J. Tranquilli-Leali or Atasoy flap: An anatomical cadaveric study. *J. Plast. Reconstr. Aesthet. Surg.* **2010**, *63*, 681–685. [CrossRef] [PubMed]
14. Lemmon, J.A.; Janis, J.E.; Rohrich, R.J. Soft-tissue injuries of the fingertip: Methods of evaluation and treatment. An Algorithmic Approach. *Plast. Reconstr. Surg.* **2008**, *122*, 105e–117e. [CrossRef]
15. Sebastin, S.J.; Mendoza, R.T.; Chong, A.K.S.; Peng, Y.P.; Ono, S.; Chung, K.C.; Lim, A.Y.T. Application of the dorsal metacarpal artery perforator flap for resurfacing soft-tissue defects proximal to the fingertip. *Plast. Reconstr. Surg.* **2011**, *128*, 166e–178e. [CrossRef]
16. Behan, F.C. The keystone design perforator island flap in reconstructive surgery. *ANZ J. Surg.* **2003**, *73*, 112–120. [CrossRef]
17. Yoon, C.S.; Kim, H.B.; Kim, Y.K.; Kim, H.; Kim, K.N. Relaxed skin tension line–oriented keystone–designed perforator island flaps considering the facial aesthetic unit concept for the coverage of small to moderate facial defects. *Medicine* **2019**, *98*, e14167. [CrossRef]
18. Yoon, C.S.; Kim, H.B.; Kim, Y.K.; Kim, H.; Kim, K.N. Keystone-design perforator island flaps for the management of complicated epidermoid cysts on the back. *Sci. Rep.* **2019**, *9*, 14699. [CrossRef]
19. Gupta, S.; Chittoria, R.K.; Chavan, V.; Aggarwal, A.; Reddy, C.L.; Mohan, P.B.; Shijina, K.; Pathan, I. Role of keystone flap in finger reconstruction. *Clin. Surg. J.* **2019**, *2*, 11–15.
20. Rajabtork Zadeh, O.; Rizzo, M.I.; Monarca, C. The versatility of keystone flap: Reconstructive option in ring finger. *Plast. Reconstr. Surg. Glob. Open.* **2020**, *8*, e2526. [CrossRef]
21. Lee, D.H.; Mignemi, M.E.; Crosby, S.N. Fingertip injuries: An update on management. *J. Am. Acad. Orthop. Surg.* **2013**, *21*, 756–766. [CrossRef] [PubMed]

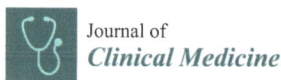
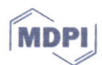

Article

Objective Skin Quality Assessment after Reconstructive Procedures for Facial Skin Defects

Dinko Martinovic [1,2], Slaven Lupi-Ferandin [1], Daria Tokic [3], Mislav Usljebrka [1], Andrija Rados [1], Ante Pojatina [1], Sanja Kadic [1], Ema Puizina [1], Ante Mihovilovic [1], Marko Kumric [2], Marino Vilovic [2], Dario Leskur [4] and Josko Bozic [2,*]

[1] Department of Maxillofacial Surgery, University Hospital of Split, 21000 Split, Croatia; dmartinovic@kbsplit.hr (D.M.); slupi@mefst.hr (S.L.-F.); musljebrka@kbsplit.hr (M.U.); arados@kbsplit.hr (A.R.); apojatina@kbsplit.hr (A.P.); skadic@kbsplit.hr (S.K.); epuizina@kbsplit.hr (E.P.); amihovilovic@kbsplit.hr (A.M.)
[2] Department of Pathophysiology, University of Split School of Medicine, 21000 Split, Croatia; marko.kumric@mefst.hr (M.K.); marino.vilovic@mefst.hr (M.V.)
[3] Department of Anesthesiology and Intensive Care, University Hospital of Split, 21000 Split, Croatia; dtokic@kbsplit.hr
[4] Department of Pharmacy, University of Split Schwool of Medicine, 21000 Split, Croatia; dario.leskur@mefst.hr
* Correspondence: josko.bozic@mefst.hr; Tel.: +385-21-557-871; Fax: +385-21-557-905

Abstract: Local random skin flaps and skin grafts are everyday surgical techniques used to reconstruct skin defects. Although their clinical advantages and disadvantages are well known, there are still uncertainties with respect to their long-term results. Hence, the aim of this study was to evaluate outcomes more than one-year post operatively using objective measurement devices. The study included 31 facial defects reconstructed with local random flap, 30 facial defects reconstructed with split-thickness skin grafts (STSGs) and 30 facial defects reconstructed with full-thickness skin grafts (FTSGs). Skin quality was objectively evaluated using MP6 noninvasive probes (Courage + Khazaka GmbH, Cologne, Germany), which measure melanin count, erythema, hydration, sebum, friction and transepidermal water loss. The results showed that there were no significant differences in melanin count, erythema, hydration, sebum level, friction value and transepidermal water loss (TEWL) between the site reconstructed with random local flaps and the same site on the healthy contralateral side of the face. However, both FTSGs and STSGs showed significantly higher levels in terms of TEWL and erythema, whereas the levels of hydration, sebum and friction were significantly lower compared to the healthy contralateral side. Moreover, STSGs resulted in a significant difference in melanin count. These findings imply that the complex pathophysiology of the wound-healing process possibly results in better skin-quality outcomes for random local flaps than skin autografts. Consequently, this suggests that random local flaps should be implemented whenever possible for the reconstruction of facial region defects.

Keywords: skin flap; skin graft; skin quality; reconstructive surgery; facial surgery

Citation: Martinovic, D.; Lupi-Ferandin, S.; Tokic, D.; Usljebrka, M.; Rados, A.; Pojatina, A.; Kadic, S.; Puizina, E.; Mihovilovic, A.; Kumric, M.; et al. Objective Skin Quality Assessment after Reconstructive Procedures for Facial Skin Defects. *J. Clin. Med.* 2022, 11, 4471. https://doi.org/10.3390/jcm11154471

Academic Editor: Giovanni Salzano

Received: 8 July 2022
Accepted: 28 July 2022
Published: 31 July 2022

Publisher's Note: MDPI stays neutral with regard to jurisdictional claims in published maps and institutional affiliations.

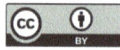

Copyright: © 2022 by the authors. Licensee MDPI, Basel, Switzerland. This article is an open access article distributed under the terms and conditions of the Creative Commons Attribution (CC BY) license (https://creativecommons.org/licenses/by/4.0/).

1. Introduction

Reconstruction of skin defects is one of the oldest surgical techniques most commonly performed after traumatic injuries or oncological excisions. Apart from primary closure and secondary healing, there is a broad range of possible reconstruction methods, such as skin autografts, local flaps, distant/regional flaps, and microvascular free tissue transfer [1–3]. The facial region is especially sensitive with respect to the selection of an appropriate reconstruction method to provide functional and aesthetically pleasing results. Whereas larger and profounder defects that affect several types of tissues are usually reconstructed using distant and regional flaps or more modern techniques, such as free flaps, somewhat smaller and superficial defects can be reconstructed using random local flaps or skin autografts [4,5].

Skin autografts are autotransplants from a patient's donor site to the defect site. Depending on the thickness, they can be divided into split-thickness skin grafts (STSGs) and full-thickness skin grafts (FTSGs) [6,7]. STSGs involve the epidermis and part of the underlying dermis, whereas FTSGs involve the epidermis and the entire dermis [8]. FTSG is usually chosen for small defects when the best possible aesthetic result is needed; in the facial region, FTSG is usually used for the nose, ear or eyelid. On the other hand, STSG is usually used to covering somewhat diametrically larger defects in the temporal region, forehead or the scalp. However, depending on the patient's status and the defect, both FTSGs and STSGs can be used in various regions [9]. Skin autografts do not have an initially autonomous blood supply, and in the first 48–72 h, they are bound to the absorbing transudate from the recipient site, a process called plasmatic imbibition [10]. Consequently, they can only survive on tissues such as the subcutis, periosteum, perichondrium and muscles, which can provide them with nutrients through the transudate. During the first days after grafting, the capillary buds start the revascularization phase, which should be completed within 5–7 d [11]. Then, the remodeling phase starts, wherein the graft undergoes retraction, adjustment and reinnervation [12].

Local random flaps are full-thickness skin with the subcutaneous layer sectioned and detached on all except one side (usually one lateral side); however, in certain types of flaps, the base serves as the only attachment (called the peduncle), and the flap vitality is determined by its vascularization [13–16]. After reconstruction, flaps adapt to the reduced vascularization, but over time, the blood supply increases due to the hyperplasia of the peduncle circulation and neovascularization from the wound margins [17]. Whereas arterial flaps survive with the help of a specific artery, random flaps depend on random circulation through the superficial subcutaneous layer, which is the richest in the facial region.

Both skin autografts and local random flaps are among the most commonly used reconstruction techniques in plastic surgery of the facial region. However, there are still some uncertainties with respect to their healing processes, especially regarding their long-term results. Most relevant data regarding the advantages and disadvantages of these methods were established in the 20th century [18]. According to the principle of reconstruction of "the same from the same", local random flaps should be more aesthetically pleasant than skin autografts for the facial region [19]. Furthermore, discoloration of the recipient site is a considered a major weakness of skin autografts compared local random flaps [20]. Moreover, local random flaps usually produce a lesser degree of scaring due to the absence of a strong secondary contraction, which is prominent in skin autografts, especially STSGs. Furthermore, skin flaps and FTSGs involve all skin appendages, whereas STSGs do not. However, none of these established advantages and disadvantages have been evaluated directly on the skin using an objective instrument after the wound-healing remodeling phase (>year after the procedure).

Hence, the primary aim of this study was to evaluate objective skin quality parameters in the facial region following reconstruction with local random flaps, FTSGs and STSGs. The secondary goal was to evaluate these same objective parameters on the healthy contralateral side of the face for comparison with the reconstructed area and to compare their differences (Δ) between the aforementioned reconstruction methods.

2. Materials and Methods

2.1. Study Design and Ethical Considerations

This cross-sectional study was performed at the Department of Maxillofacial Surgery, University Hospital of Split, during the time period from June 2021 to January 2022.

All subjects were informed about the purpose and procedures of the study in a timely manner, and they all signed an informed consent to participate. The study was approved by the Ethics Committee of the University Hospital of Split and conducted in accordance with the latest version of the Declaration of Helsinki.

2.2. Subjects

The study included 31 facial defects reconstructed with local random flap, 30 facial defects reconstructed with STSGs and 30 facial defects reconstructed with FTSGs. Participants were recruited to the study during control check-ups. All included participants underwent an operation due to basal cell carcinoma (BCC) or squamous cell carcinoma (SCC). Furthermore, all three reconstructive procedures were conducted at the Department of Maxillofacial Surgery, University Hospital of Split, according to the standard surgical protocols and guidelines. Our institution prefers local skin flaps over skin autografts for facial reconstruction. Indications for use of FTSGs were the nasal and eyelid areas, whereas the indication for use of STSGs was diametrically larger defects (>40 mm) in the frontotemporal and forehead areas. However, these indications are individually dependent on the patient's age, status and skin elasticity.

The inclusion criteria for participants were age of 18–90 years, >1 year since reconstruction, no postoperative complications and a healthy contralateral side of the face. According to most authors, skin healing and remodeling is completed one year after reconstruction. Additionally, only patients with FTSGs from supraclavicular donor sites were included, as well as only STSGs from upper-arm donor sites (0.4 mm thickness during harvest).

Exclusion criteria were paramedial location of the reconstructed defect, recidivism of the malignancy, re-excision of the reconstructed site, other active malignant diseases, diabetes mellitus, chronic dermatological diseases, smoking, excessive alcohol consumption and psychiatric diseases. Prior to inclusion, all subjects underwent a detailed physical examination and meticulous inspection of their anamnestic data.

2.3. Objective Skin Assessment

Skin quality was objectively evaluated by the same experienced investigator using an MP6 skin quality assessment instrument (Courage + Khazaka GmbH, Cologne, Germany). The instrument assesses several skin qualities using noninvasive probes. Transepidermal water loss (TEWL) was assessed as an objective sign of skin barrier function using a Tewameter® TM 300 instrument. Skin hydration was assessed using a Corneometer® CM 825. The amount of erythema and melanin was measured using a Mexameter® MX 18. Skin friction was estimated using a Frictiometer® FR 700. Sebum was measured using a Sebumeter® SM 815. All probes were calibrated according to the manufacturers' instructions before study onset.

All participants underwent measurements in a room with stable conditions. Air humidity was kept at 40–55% using a Philips 3000i air humidifier (Koninklijke Philips N.V., Amsterdam, the Netherlands), and the room temperature was kept at 20–22 °C using the inbuilt hospital air conditioners. The participants were first seated in the room for 20 min to acclimate the skin to the aforementioned conditions. Participants were instructed to take a shower the morning of the measurement day and to strictly avoid using any make-up, skin creams or any other skin preparations. Probes were used to measure both the reconstructed area and the same area on the contralateral healthy side. The probes were held at a right angle and gently applied to the skin for optimal contact, and all measurements were performed three times, after which the mean value was calculated. After every participant, probes were disinfected and prepared for the next subject.

The same site on the healthy contralateral side was measured as a referent value, and to diminish the interparticipant variability, we computed the difference (Δ) between the healthy and reconstructed site (Δ = healthy site parameter—reconstructed site parameter).

Moreover, to test for possible intraobserver variability, several participants underwent objective evaluation with the probes on three (3) different days. There was no statistically significant difference between these results.

2.4. Statistical Analyses and Sample Size Calculation

All data analyses were performed using MedCalc statistical software (MedCalc Software, version 20.110, Ostend, Belgium). Qualitative variables are presented as whole numbers and percentages. Continuous quantitative data are presented as mean ± standard deviation, whereas non-continuous data are presented as median and interquartile range. The normality of the data distribution was estimated using the Kolmogorov–Smirnov test. A chi-square test was used for comparison of categorical variables. A student's t-test was used for comparison of parametric variables, whereas a Mann–Whitney U test was used for comparison of non-parametric variables. One-way analysis of variance (ANOVA) with post hoc Tukey's test was used for comparison of parametric variables between groups, whereas Kruskal–Wallis test with post hoc Dunn's test was used for comparison of non-parametric variables between groups. The level of statistical significance was set $p < 0.05$.

Sample size was analyzed using the data from a pilot study on 15 randomly selected subjects from the patient population (5 patients with random flaps, 5 patients with FTSGs and 5 patients with STSGs). Melanin count difference (Δ), which was one the main outcomes of the study, was used for the calculation. In random flap patients, the mean melanin Δ was 2.0 ± 6.0 AU, whereas in FTSG patients, it was -6.1 ± 7.0 AU, and in STSG patients, it was -29.0 ± 15 AU. With a type I error of 0.05 and a power of 90%, the required sample size was 15 participants per group.

3. Results

There were 50 (55.0%) male and 41 (45.0%) female participants included, and the mean age of the study population was 78.6 ± 8.3 years. With respect to the defect diameter, STSGs had the largest size, with a significant difference relative to the other two groups ($p < 0.001$). There were no other significant differences between the three groups with respect to the anthropometric and clinical characteristics (Table 1).

Table 1. Anthropometric and clinical characteristics of the study sample.

Parameter	Study Population (N = 93)	Flaps (N = 31)	FTSGs (N = 30)	STSGs (N = 30)	p
Male gender (N,%)	51 (55.0)	17 (54.8)	18 (60.0)	16 (53.3)	0.861 *
Age (years)	78.6 ± 8.3	76.5 ± 7.0	79.3 ± 9.0	79.8 ± 8.6	0.243 †
Body height (cm)	179.1 ± 10.8	178.2 ± 9.6	177.2 ± 7.5	181.0 ± 11.1	0.136 †
Body mass (kg)	78.2 ± 8.9	77.6 ± 8.7	76.5 ± 10.9	80.4 ± 6.3	0.199 †
BMI (kg/m^2)	24.5 ± 2.7	24.7 ± 2.8	24.1 ± 2.8	24.4 ± 2.6	0.672 †
Time since the op. (mo)	32 (28–46)	34 (26–48)	36 (30–52)	30 (28–34)	0.101 ‡
BCC (N,%)	54 (58.1)	20 (64.5)	18 (60.0)	15 (50.0)	0.502 *
SCC (N,%)	39 (41.9)	11 (35.5)	12 (40.0)	15 (50.0)	
Defect diameter (mm)	32 (22–44)	25 (17–32)	29 (19–33)	49 (42–54)	<0.001 ‡

All data are presented as whole numbers (percentages), mean ± standard deviation or median (interquartile range). **Abbreviations:** FTSG—full-thickness skin graft; STSG—split-thickness skin graft; BMI—body mass index; BCC—basal cell carcinoma; SCC—squamous cell carcinoma; * chi-square; † one-way analysis of variance (ANOVA) with post hoc Tukey's test; ‡ Kruskal–Wallis test with post hoc Dunn's test.

There were no significant differences with respect to the objective skin parameters between the random local flaps and the healthy contralateral side for all tested parameters (Table 2). However, both FTSG and STSG and patients presented a significantly higher erythema level and TEWL, and both groups showed a significantly lower level of hydration, sebum and friction compared to the healthy contralateral side (Table 2). However, only STSG patients presented significantly higher melanin counts ($p < 0.001$) (Table 2).

After calculating the difference (Δ) of the skin parameters between the healthy and the reconstructed site, we compared them between the local random flaps, FTSG and STSG groups. We observed a significant difference in melanin ($H = 69.498$; $p < 0.001$), with random skin flaps resulting in the lowest difference and STSG with the highest difference (flaps: 4.0 (−3.0–7.0); FTSG: −7.0 (−10.0–−3.0); STSG: −33.0 (−43.0–−29.0)) (Figure 1). Post hoc analysis showed a significant difference between all three groups ($p < 0.05$) (Figure 1).

Table 2. Comparison of objective skin parameters between the reconstructed site and the healthy contralateral side.

Parameter	Reconstruction Site	Healthy Contralateral Side	p *
Random Skin Flap (N = 31)			
Melanin (AU)	113.0 ± 36.3	115.0 ± 37.2	0.836 *
Erythema (AU)	329 (297–343)	322 (283–362)	0.341 †
Hydration (AU)	49.1 ± 14.4	51.1 ± 14.5	0.587 *
Sebum (AU)	28.0 (21.2–56.0)	29.0 (18.0–54.0)	0.760 †
Friction (AU)	138.0 (68.0–189.0)	152.0 (77.0–200.0)	0.371 †
TEWL (g/m^2/h)	11.5 (10.4–13.3)	11.0 (9.9–13.2)	0.799 †
FTSG (N = 30)			
Melanin (AU)	82.4 ± 31.1	74.6 ± 30.3	0.319 *
Erythema (AU)	379 (288–404)	244 (187–291)	<0.001 †
Hydration (AU)	29.0 ± 13.0	36.5 ± 13.7	0.032 *
Sebum (AU)	17.0 (11.0–28.0)	28.0 (24.2–35.0)	<0.001 †
Friction (AU)	82.0 (75.0–129.0)	122.0 (91.0–185.7)	<0.035 †
TEWL (g/m^2/h)	13.0 (12.0–15.3)	10.9 (9.8–13.0)	<0.001 †
STSG (N = 30)			
Melanin (AU)	119.0 ± 28.9	83.1 ± 27.6	<0.001 *
Erythema (AU)	338 (314–396)	222 (181–289)	<0.001 †
Hydration (AU)	19.9 ± 6.3	37.9 ± 8.2	<0.001 *
Sebum (AU)	21.0 (10.0–24.0)	39.0 (41.0–72.0)	<0.001 †
Friction (AU)	81.0 (58.0–137.7)	121.1 (106.0–212.7)	<0.001 †
TEWL (g/m^2/h)	13.1 (11.8–14.2)	10.8 (9.4–12.3)	<0.001 †

All data are presented as median (IQR). **Abbreviations: FTSG**—full-thickness skin graft; **STSG**—split-thickness skin graft; **TEWL**—transepidermal water loss. * Student's *t*-test; † Mann–Whitney U test.

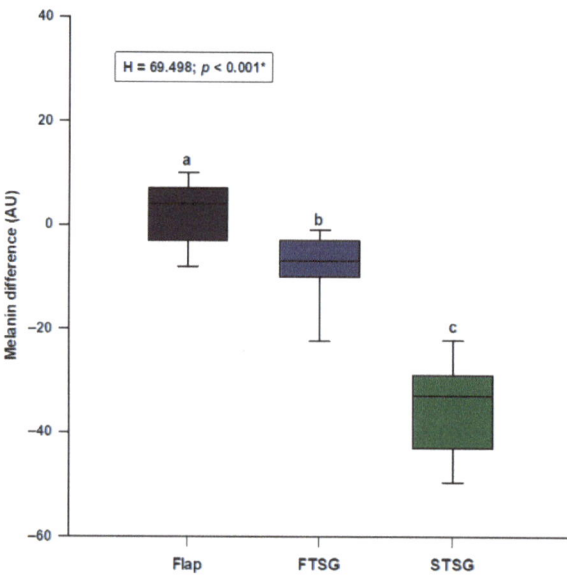

Figure 1. Comparison of the melanin difference between the random local flaps (N = 31), STSG (N = 30) and FTSG (N = 30) groups. **Abbreviations: FTSG**—full-thickness skin graft; **STSG**—split-thickness skin graft. * Kruskal–Wallis test with post hoc Dunn's test. a vs. b—$p < 0.05$; a vs. c—$p < 0.05$; b vs. c—$p < 0.05$.

We observed a statistically significant difference in erythema levels (H = 44.244; $p < 0.001$), with the random skin flap group showing the lowest difference and the STSG group presenting the highest difference (flaps: −9.0 (−14.0−−4.0); FTSG: −107.0 (−160.0−−48.0); STSG: −105.0 (−184.0−−76.0)) (Figure 2). Post hoc analysis showed a significant difference between random skin flaps and both FTSG ($p < 0.05$) and STSG ($p < 0.05$) (Figure 2).

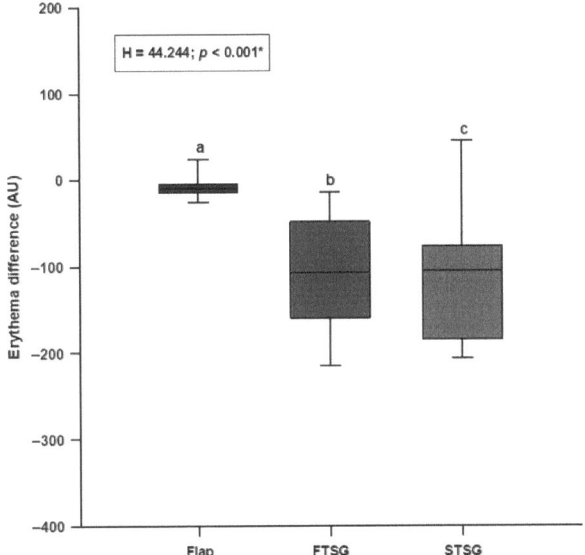

Figure 2. Comparison of the erythema difference between the random local flaps (N = 31), STSG (N = 30) and FTSG (N = 30) groups. **Abbreviations: FTSG**—full-thickness skin graft; **STSG**—split-thickness skin graft. * Kruskal–Wallis test with post hoc Dunn's test. a vs. b—$p < 0.05$; a vs. c—$p < 0.05$; b vs. c—$p > 0.05$.

We observed a statistically significant difference in hydration (H = 53.589; $p < 0.001$), with the random skin flap group showing the lowest difference and the STSG group presenting the highest difference (flaps: 1.0 (−1.0–5.0); FTSGs: 8.0 (2.0–9.0); STSGs: 18.0 (13.0–23.0)) (Figure 3). Post hoc analysis showed a significant difference between all three groups ($p < 0.05$) (Figure 3).

We observed a statistically significant difference in sebum (H = 56.315; $p < 0.001$), with the random skin flap group showing the lowest difference and the STSG group presenting the highest difference (flaps: 1.0 (−4.0–3.0); FTSGs: 8.0 (2.0–17.0); STSGs: 25.0 (20.0–42.0)) (Figure 4). Post hoc analysis showed a significant difference between all three groups ($p < 0.05$) (Figure 4).

We observed a statistically significant difference in friction (H = 14.017; $p < 0.001$), with the random skin flap group showing the lowest difference and the STSG group presenting the highest difference (flaps: 0.0 (−21.0—49.0); FTSGs: 20.0 (15.0—40.0); STSGs: 51.0 (21.0—83.0)) (Figure 5). Post hoc analysis showed a significant difference between random skin flaps and STSGs ($p < 0.05$) (Figure 5).

TEWL showed a statistically significant difference (H = 42.965; $p < 0.001$) with random skin flaps showing the lowest difference and STSGs presenting the highest difference (Flaps: −0.6 (−0.9–0.6); FTSGs: −1.8 (−2.4−−1.1); STSGs: −2.1 (−3.0−−1.2)) (Figure 6). Post hoc analysis showed a significant difference between random skin flaps and both the FTSG ($p < 0.05$) and STSG ($p < 0.05$) groups (Figure 6).

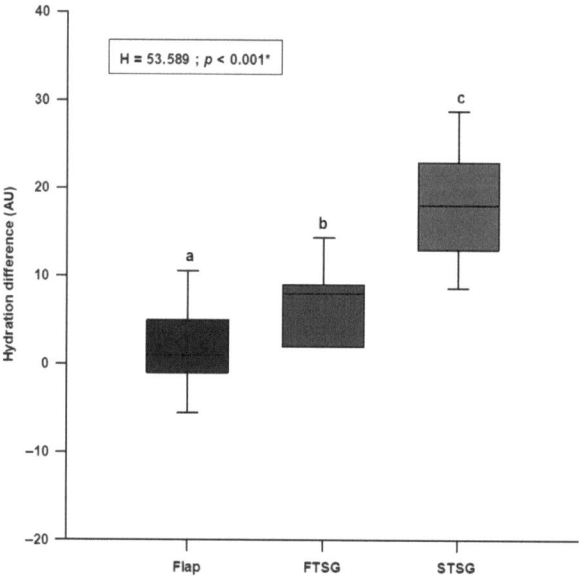

Figure 3. Comparison of the hydration difference between the random local flaps (N = 31), STSG (N = 30) and FTSG (N = 30) groups. **Abbreviations: FTSG**—full–thickness skin graft; **STSG**—split-thickness skin graft. * Kruskal–Wallis test with post hoc Dunn's test. a vs. b—$p < 0.05$; a vs. c—$p < 0.05$; b vs. c—$p < 0.05$.

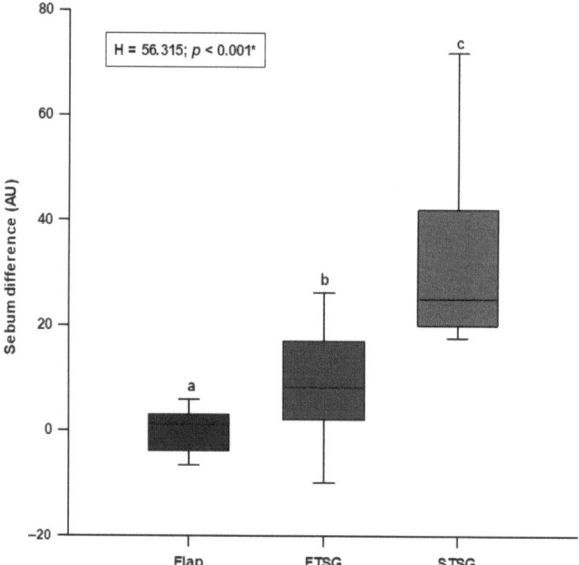

Figure 4. Comparison of the sebum difference between the random local flaps (N = 31), STSG (N = 30) and FTSG (N = 30) groups. **Abbreviation: FTSG**—full-thickness skin graft; **STSG**—split-thickness skin graft. * Kruskal–Wallis test with post hoc Dunn's test. a vs. b—$p < 0.05$; a vs. c—$p < 0.05$; b vs. c—$p < 0.05$.

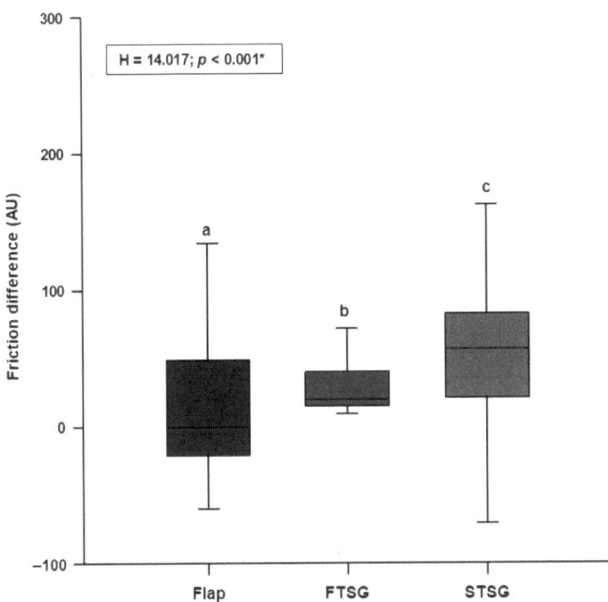

Figure 5. Comparison of the friction difference between the random local flaps (N = 31), STSGs (N = 30) and FTSGs (N = 30). **Abbreviation: FTSG**—full-thickness skin graft; **STSG**—split-thickness skin graft. * Kruskal–Wallis test with post hoc Dunn's test. a vs. b—$p > 0.05$. a vs. c—$p < 0.05$. b vs. c—$p > 0.05$.

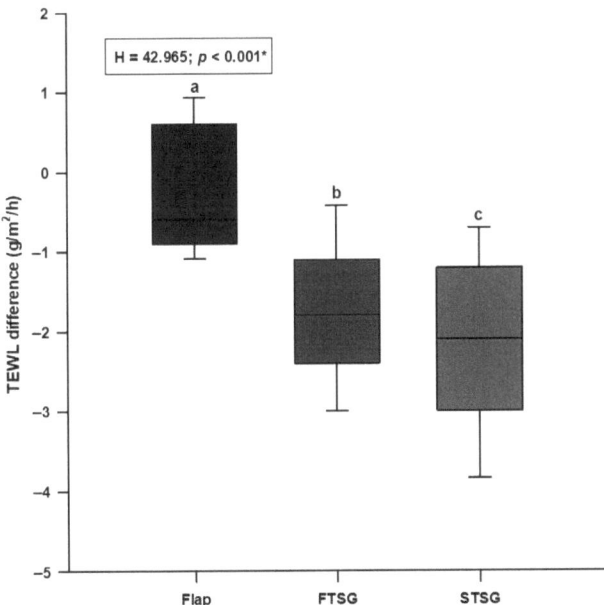

Figure 6. Comparison of the TEWL difference between the random local flaps (N = 31), STSG (N = 30) and FTSG (N = 30) groups. **Abbreviations: FTSG**—full-thickness skin graft; **STSG**—split-thickness skin graft; **TEWL**—transepidermal water loss. * Kruskal–Wallis test with post hoc Dunn's test. a vs. b—$p < 0.05$; a vs. c—$p < 0.05$; b vs. c—$p > 0.05$.

4. Discussion

The results of this study showed that there were no significant differences in melanin count, erythema, hydration, sebum level, friction value and TEWL between the site reconstructed with random local flaps and the same site on the healthy contralateral side of the face. However, both the FTSG and STSG groups had significantly higher levels of TEWL and erythema, whereas hydration, sebum and friction levels were significantly lower compared to the healthy contralateral side. The STSG group also had higher melanin counts. With respect to differences (Δ) between the healthy and reconstructed site, the results showed a significant difference between the three reconstruction methods in all parameters. Moreover, post hoc analyses revealed that the random local flaps group had the lowest Δ, whereas the STSG group had the highest Δ regarding all evaluated skin quality parameters. Based on an extensive search of the available literature, we concluded that this is the first study to objectively compare skin quality between local random flaps, FTSG and STSG.

The results of our objective skin evaluations are partially in line with the recognized advantages and disadvantages of local flaps, FTSG and STSG. Discoloration is one of the main aesthetic disadvantages of FTSG and STSG for facial reconstruction [21,22]. However, FTSG causes a lesser degree of discoloration than STSG when harvested from the head and neck regions, such as the supraclavicular, retroauricular or scalp regions. Although FTSG still results in a certain degree of discoloration in comparison to healthy facial skin, our results showed that there was no statistically significant difference. Whereas some authors have mentioned hypopigmentation as a possible skin graft outcome, most agree that hyperpigmentation is the most frequently exhibited trait; however, the pathophysiology behind this phenomenon is still unclear. [23,24]. Whereas it seems that the grafted skin displays a higher melanin count compared to healthy skin, a study by Tsukada et al. showed that histologically, the melanocyte count was much lower in the skin graft group [25]. The proposed explanation for this paradox is that the contraction of the graft could lead to a closer approximation of melanin in the skin [26].

The contraction of has been skin grafts was well-established in numerous studies [27,28]. Whereas primary graft contraction occurs immediately after the harvest due to the passive recoil of the elastin fibers, secondary contraction occurs over time after the reconstruction due to myofibroblasts in the wound bed [28]. FTSG results in greater primary contraction owing it to the larger amount of dermis, whereas STSG results in greater secondary contraction owing it to the lesser amount of dermis, which consequently increases susceptibility to myofibroblast pulling [27]. As mentioned previously, contracture is the possible cause of skin graft hyperpigmentation, and it could also possibly influence the friction quality of the skin. Our results showed that the friction value is lowest in the STSG group and somewhat higher in FTSG group, whereas the friction was most similar to that of healthy skin in the local flaps group. These results are contrary to those reported in a study conducted on finger pads, which showed that even a small degree of tangential skin stretch, a trait equivalent to contraction, resulted in increased perceived friction [29]. Moreover, this could be especially interesting regarding our results indicating that skin grafts resulted in significantly lower hydration compared to healthy skin. It is well-established that skin hydration, which is provided by the stratum corneum, is one of the main factors that contribute to a higher skin friction value [30,31]. It is possible that the hydration from stratum corneum plays a greater role in skin friction than contraction similar to tangential stretch. Nevertheless, this hypothesis needs to be addressed in future studies.

As TEWL is one of the most important indicators of skin barrier function, it is an important and interesting subject with respect to skin grafts. Our results showed significantly higher TEWL in both the FTSG and STSG groups compared to the healthy side. Some of our results are contrary to those reported in a study conducted by Kim et al. wherein objective measurements were used to follow-up skin changes in STSG patients [26]. Their study showed that although there were paradoxical dynamics during months of follow-up, one year after the procedure, STSG patients did not show any statistically significant change in skin function, although TEWL and epidermal hydration levels were somewhat reduced. Another interesting point of view is presented in a study by Suetake et al., who found that keloid and hypertrophic scars have higher TEWL levels than normal skin subsequent to aberrations of the stratum corneum [32]. Although keloids and hypertrophic scars have different pathophysiological mechanisms than skin grafts, it is possible that they both exhibit functional abnormalities of the stratum corneum.

Another result of this study that should be highlighted is the lower sebum levels found in skin autografts, most prominently in STSG patients. The dermis contains connective tissue and skin appendages, such as sebaceous glands, hair follicles and sweat glands. Although sebaceous glands are seated in the dermis, hair follicles and sweat glands extend into subcutaneous fat. Studies have shown that transplanted appendages survive in skin grafts; however, because only a part of the dermis is included, STSG patients often have functionally deficient sebaceous glands, sweat glands and hair follicles [33]. Sebum also plays an important role as a skin barrier facilitator. A study conducted on radiation-induced skin injury showed that the atrophy of sebaceous glands had a considerable impact on TEWL and skin hydration [34].

There are several limitations to our study. First of all, we were not able to eliminate all of the confounding effects, and the cross-sectional design prohibited making any causal conclusions. Moreover, our sample size was relatively small, and the study was conducted in a single center. Additionally, the instrument used for objective skin quality assessments has a noted interobserver variability. We mitigated this limitation by using only one experienced investigator for all instrumental evaluations.

5. Conclusions

Our results showed that after the remodeling phase (>1 year postoperative), random local skin flaps resulted in significantly better skin quality than STSG and FTSG. These findings imply that the complex pathophysiology of the wound-healing process possibly results in better skin quality outcomes for random local flaps than skin autografts. Moreover, these outcomes suggest that random local flaps should be implemented in the reconstruction of the facial region defects when permitted by the reconstruction site and size of defect. However, larger multicentric, longitudinal studies are needed to further address our findings.

Author Contributions: Conceptualization, D.M., S.L.-F., D.T., M.U., M.V. and J.B.; methodology, D.M., S.L.-F., D.T., M.V., D.L. and J.B.; software, D.M., A.R., A.P., S.K., E.P. and A.M.; validation, D.M., D.T., E.P., A.M., M.K., M.V. and D.L.; formal analysis, D.M., D.T., M.U., A.R., A.P. and S.K.; investigation, D.M., M.U., A.R. and A.P.; resources, D.M., M.V. and D.L.; data curation, D.M., D.T., M.U., E.P., M.K., M.V. and D.L.; writing—original draft preparation, D.M., D.T., S.K. and M.K.; writing—review and editing, D.M., D.T. and M.K.; visualization, D.M., M.U., A.R., A.P., E.P. and A.M.; supervision, D.M., S.L.-F., D.L. and J.B.; project administration, D.M., S.L.-F., D.L. and J.B.; funding acquisition, S.L.-F. and J.B. All authors have read and agreed to the published version of the manuscript.

Funding: This research received no external funding.

Institutional Review Board Statement: The study was conducted in accordance with the Declaration of Helsinki and approved by the Ethics Committee of the University Hospital of Split (protocol code: 500-03/21-01/75; date of approval: 4 May 2021).

Informed Consent Statement: Informed consent was obtained from all subjects involved in the study.

Data Availability Statement: All data sets are available upon request to the corresponding author.

Conflicts of Interest: The authors declare no conflict of interest.

References

1. Shimizu, R.; Kishi, K. Skin graft. *Plast. Surg. Int.* **2012**, *2012*, 563493. [CrossRef]
2. Schultz, T.A.; Cunningham, K.; Bailey, J.S. Basic flap design. *Oral Maxillofac. Surg. Clin.* **2014**, *26*, 277–303. [CrossRef] [PubMed]
3. Wolff, K.D. New aspects in free flap surgery: Mini-perforator flaps and extracorporeal flap perfusion. *J. Stomatol. Oral Maxillofac. Surg.* **2017**, *118*, 238–241. [CrossRef] [PubMed]
4. Simman, R. Wound closure and the reconstructive ladder in plastic surgery. *J. Am. Coll. Certif. Wound Spec.* **2009**, *1*, 6–11. [CrossRef] [PubMed]
5. Mégevand, V.; Suva, D.; Mohamad, M.; Hannouche, D.; Kalbermatten, D.F.; Oranges, C.M. Muscle vs. fasciocutaneous microvascular free flaps for lower limb reconstruction: A meta-analysis of comparative studies. *J. Clin. Med.* **2022**, *11*, 1557. [CrossRef] [PubMed]
6. Adams, D.C.; Ramsey, M.L. Grafts in dermatologic surgery: Review and update on full- and split-thickness skin grafts, free cartilage grafts, and composite grafts. *Derm. Surg.* **2005**, *31*, 1055–1067. [CrossRef] [PubMed]
7. Straub, A.; Brands, R.; Borgmann, A.; Vollmer, A.; Hohm, J.; Linz, C.; Müller-Richter, U.; Kübler, A.C.; Hartmann, S. Free Skin Grafting to reconstruct donor sites after radial forearm flap harvesting: A prospective study with platelet-rich fibrin (PRF). *J. Clin. Med.* **2022**, *11*, 3506. [CrossRef]
8. Sapino, G.; Lanz, L.; Roesti, A.; Guillier, D.; Deglise, S.; De Santis, G.; Raffoul, W.; di Summa, P. One-stage coverage of leg region defects with STSG combined with VAC dressing improves early patient mobilisation and graft take: A comparative study. *J. Clin. Med.* **2022**, *11*, 3305. [CrossRef] [PubMed]
9. Zilinsky, I.; Farber, N.; Weissman, O.; Israeli, H.; Haik, J.; Domniz, N.; Winkler, E. Defying consensus: Correct sizing of full-thickness skin grafts. *J. Drugs Dermatol.* **2012**, *11*, 520–523. [PubMed]
10. Andreassi, A.; Bilenchi, R.; Biagioli, M.; D'Aniello, C. Classification and pathophysiology of skin grafts. *Clin. Dermatol.* **2005**, *23*, 332–337. [CrossRef] [PubMed]
11. Gould, D.J.; Reece, G.P. Skin graft vascular maturation and remodeling: A multifractal approach to morphological quantification. *Microcirculation* **2012**, *19*, 652–663. [CrossRef]
12. Prohaska, J.; Cook, C. Skin Grafting. In *StatPearls*; StatPearls Publishing: St. Petersburg, FL, USA, 2022.
13. Rao, J.K.; Shende, K.S. Overview of local flaps of the face for reconstruction of cutaneous malignancies: Single institutional experience of seventy cases. *J. Cutan. Aesthetic Surg.* **2016**, *9*, 220–225. [CrossRef]
14. Maciel-Miranda, A.; Morris, S.F.; Hallock, G.G. Local flaps, including pedicled perforator flaps: Anatomy, technique, and applications. *Plast. Reconstr. Surg.* **2013**, *131*, 896e–911e. [CrossRef]
15. Salibian, A.A.; Zide, B.M. Elegance in upper lip reconstruction. *Plast. Reconstr. Surg.* **2019**, *143*, 572–582. [CrossRef]
16. Mohan, A.T.; Sur, Y.J.; Zhu, L.; Morsy, M.; Wu, P.S.; Moran, S.L.; Mardini, S.; Saint-Cyr, M. The concepts of propeller, perforator, keystone, and other local flaps and their role in the evolution of reconstruction. *Plast. Reconstr. Surg.* **2016**, *138*, 710e–729e. [CrossRef]
17. Wu, Z.J.; Ibrahim, M.M.; Sergesketter, A.R.; Schweller, R.M.; Phillips, B.T.; Klitzman, B. The influence of topical vasodilator-induced pharmacologic delay on cutaneous flap viability and vascular remodeling. *Plast. Reconstr. Surg.* **2022**, *149*, 629–637. [CrossRef]
18. Kohlhauser, M.; Luze, H.; Nischwitz, S.P.; Kamolz, L.P. Historical evolution of skin grafting-a journey through time. *Medicina* **2021**, *57*, 348. [CrossRef]
19. Hallock, G.G.; Morris, S.F. Skin grafts and local flaps. *Plast. Reconstr. Surg.* **2011**, *127*, 5e–22e. [CrossRef]
20. Zhang, A.Y.; Meine, J.G. Flaps and grafts reconstruction. *Dermatol. Clin.* **2011**, *29*, 217–230. [CrossRef]
21. Matsumoto, K.; Robb, E.; Warden, G.; Nordlund, J. Hyperpigmentation of human skin grafted on to athymic nude mice: Immunohistochemical study. *Br. J. Dermatol.* **1996**, *135*, 412–418. [CrossRef] [PubMed]
22. Eskandarlou, M.; Taghipour, M. Outcome of comparison between Partial thickness skin graft harvesting from scalp and lower limb for scalp defect: A clinical trial study. *World J. Plast. Surg.* **2021**, *10*, 25–32. [CrossRef]
23. Weathers, W.M.; Bhadkamkar, M.; Wolfswinkel, E.M.; Thornton, J.F. Full-thickness skin grafting in nasal reconstruction. *Semin. Plast. Surg.* **2013**, *27*, 90–95. [CrossRef] [PubMed]
24. Kang, X.L.; Shen, H. Pigmentation of skin graft is improved by cryopreservation of human skin with trehalose. *J. Oral. Maxillofac. Surg.* **2012**, *70*, 1464–1472. [CrossRef] [PubMed]
25. Tsukada, S. Studies on the pigmentation of skin grafts: The ultrastructure of epidermal melanoxytes. *Plast. Reconstr. Surg.* **1977**, *59*, 98–106. [CrossRef]
26. Kim, Y.J.; Kim, M.Y.; Lee, P.K.; Kim, H.O.; Park, Y.M. Evaluation of natural change of skin function in split-thickness skin grafts by noninvasive bioengineering methods. *Dermatol. Surg.* **2006**, *32*, 1358–1363.
27. Harrison, C.A.; MacNeil, S. The mechanism of skin graft contraction: An update on current research and potential future therapies. *Burns* **2008**, *34*, 153–163. [CrossRef] [PubMed]
28. Stekelenburg, C.M.; Simons, J.M.; Tuinebreijer, W.E.; van Zuijlen, P.P. Analyzing contraction of full thickness skin grafts in time: Choosing the donor site does matter. *Burns* **2016**, *42*, 1471–1476. [CrossRef] [PubMed]
29. Provancher, W.R.; Sylvester, N.D. Fingerpad skin stretch increases the perception of virtual friction. *IEEE Trans. Haptics.* **2009**, *2*, 212–223. [CrossRef] [PubMed]

30. Zhu, Y.H.; Song, S.P.; Luo, W.; Elias, P.M.; Man, M.Q. Characterization of skin friction coefficient, and relationship to stratum corneum hydration in a normal Chinese population. *Ski. Pharm. Physiol* **2011**, *24*, 81–86. [CrossRef] [PubMed]
31. Leyva-Mendivil, M.F.; Lengiewicz, J.; Page, A.; Bressloff, N.W.; Limbert, G. Skin microstructure is a key contributor to its friction behaviour. *Tribol. Lett.* **2017**, *65*, 12. [CrossRef]
32. Suetake, T.; Sasai, S.; Zhen, Y.X.; Ohi, T.; Tagami, H. Functional analyses of the stratum corneum in scars. Sequential studies after injury and comparison among keloids, hypertrophic scars, and atrophic scars. *Arch. Dermatol.* **1996**, *132*, 1453–1458. [CrossRef] [PubMed]
33. Matsuo, S.; Kurisaki, A.; Sugino, H.; Hashimoto, I.; Nakanishi, H. Analysis of skin graft survival using green fluorescent protein transgenic mice. *J. Med. Investg.* **2007**, *54*, 267–275. [CrossRef] [PubMed]
34. Jang, H.; Myung, H.; Lee, J.; Myung, J.K.; Jang, W.-S.; Lee, S.-J.; Bae, C.-H.; Kim, H.; Park, S.; Shim, S. Impaired skin barrier due to sebaceous gland atrophy in the latent stage of radiation-induced skin injury: Application of non-invasive diagnostic methods. *Int. J. Mol. Sci.* **2018**, *19*, 185. [CrossRef] [PubMed]

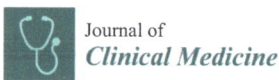 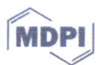

Article

Preliminary Single-Center Experience of Bromelain-Based Eschar Removal in Children with Mixed Deep Dermal and Full Thickness Burns

Tomasz Korzeniowski [1,2,*], Ewelina Grywalska [3], Jerzy Strużyna [2,4], Magdalena Bugaj-Tobiasz [2], Agnieszka Surowiecka [2], Izabela Korona-Główniak [5], Magdalena Staśkiewicz [6] and Kamil Torres [1]

[1] Chair and Department of Didactics and Medical Simulation, Medical University of Lublin, 20-093 Lublin, Poland
[2] East Center of Burns Treatment and Reconstructive Surgery, 21-010 Leczna, Poland
[3] Department of Experimental Immunology, Medical University of Lublin, 20-093 Lublin, Poland
[4] Chair and Department of Plastic, Reconstructive Surgery and Burn Treatment, Medical University of Lublin, 20-093 Lublin, Poland
[5] Department of Pharmaceutical Microbiology, Medical University of Lublin, 20-093 Lublin, Poland
[6] Center for Innovation and Accreditation, Medical University of Lublin, 20-093 Lublin, Poland
* Correspondence: t.korzeniowski@gmail.com

Abstract: Introduction: Early eschar removal is the standard management of burns. The goal is to remove all of the necrotic tissue and render the wound suitable for healing or skin grafting. The enzymatic debridement of burn wounds allows for minimally invasive removal of burn eschar. The aim of the study was to describe and compare the demographic characteristics, surgical treatment and outcomes of patients treated with Nexobrid® with patients who had standard surgical excision. Material and Methods: A retrospective review was conducted on children who underwent enzymatic debridement. The study group was compared with children treated with the standard of care (SoC). Results: Twelve children (mean age 8 years, range 3 to 15 years) with mixed deep dermal and full thickness burn wounds were treated with Nexobrid®. The mean size of the burns was 29% TBSA. The median percentage TBSA debrided using Nexobrid® was 15% (range 2–27%). In a clinical assessment, enzymatic debridement was effective in removing dead tissue in a single application. No adverse reaction to Nexobrid® and serious complications after enzymatic procedure were recorded in the study group. The estimated relative risk of the need for reconstructive procedures decreases 3.5 times for the study group (RR 3.5, 95%CI 0.9–13.5, $p = 0.089$). Conclusion: The bromelain-based enzymatic method offers a good and safe debridement option to improve the treatment and life quality of children with severe burns. The main outcome of interest was the number of reconstructive procedures due to scar contractures, which was reduced in the group treated enzymatically compared to the SoC-treated children.

Keywords: wound healing; burns; enzymatic debridement

Citation: Korzeniowski, T.; Grywalska, E.; Strużyna, J.; Bugaj-Tobiasz, M.; Surowiecka, A.; Korona-Główniak, I.; Staśkiewicz, M.; Torres, K. Preliminary Single-Center Experience of Bromelain-Based Eschar Removal in Children with Mixed Deep Dermal and Full Thickness Burns. *J. Clin. Med.* **2022**, *11*, 4800. https://doi.org/10.3390/jcm11164800

Academic Editors: Giovanni Salzano and Roberto Cuomo

Received: 16 July 2022
Accepted: 15 August 2022
Published: 17 August 2022

Publisher's Note: MDPI stays neutral with regard to jurisdictional claims in published maps and institutional affiliations.

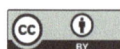

Copyright: © 2022 by the authors. Licensee MDPI, Basel, Switzerland. This article is an open access article distributed under the terms and conditions of the Creative Commons Attribution (CC BY) license (https://creativecommons.org/licenses/by/4.0/).

1. Introduction

Early burn wound debridement is regarded as the major factor in reducing invasive burn infection and improving survival [1]. Infection is the leading cause of death in both the adults and children who survive the initial resuscitation through burn shock. Following thermal injury, the skin's impaired barrier function, combined with the anatomical features of pediatric skin, make children more susceptible to inflammation and infection. As long as the necrotic tissue is present, the risk of infection persists. Early wound excision and coverage have become the key clinical strategy to improve burn wound care [2–4]. The decision to remove the eschar is critical. The most important decision-making process is therefore deciding when to operate, and at what depth to debride the wound for the optimal healing and recovery. Debridement within the first 24 h after injury significantly decreases the bacterial colonization and subsequent infection in pediatric burn patients [5,6]. The standard of care is surgical necrectomy, using sharp excision. However, the sacrifice with this method is the unintentional removal of healthy, viable tissue along with the intentional removal of the necrotic tissue. The principal drawback of the fascia excision is that it may create a considerable contour deformity. The non-excisional eschar removal methods include abrasion technique, hydro-surgery and enzymatic debridement [7]. The latter, with the use of Nexobrid® rich in bromelain-based enzyme agents, is growing in popularity. The enzymatic debridement of burn wounds allows for the minimally invasive removal of necrotic tissue. Recent studies confirm the efficacy, selectivity and safety of this method [8,9]. This study aimed to describe and compare the demographic characteristics, surgical treatment and outcomes of the patients treated with Nexobrid® with patients who had standard surgical excision.

2. Material and Methods

A retrospective chart review of the children who underwent enzymatic debridement or surgical necrectomy at the East Centre of Burns Treatment and Reconstructive Surgery in Leczna (Poland) was conducted. These were all pediatric patients with mixed deep dermal and full thickness burns treated in 2015–2020.

The enzymatic debridement was performed using Nexobrid® (eschar-specific removal agent) comprising a mixture of proteolytic enzymes and bromelain (derived from the pineapple stem), according to the following protocol: thoroughly cleaning the wound with antiseptic solution and removal of dead epidermis; soaking with moisturizing dressing for 2 h; preparing and applying the Nexobrid® mixture to the wound along with an occlusive dressing for 4 h; removing dissolved eschar and product remnants via scraping; wet to dry dressing with polyhexanide solution for at least 2 h.

The eschar removal procedure using Nexobrid® was performed on the first day or no later than the second day after injury, under opiate or general anesthesia in the operating theatre. The vital parameters of all of the children were monitored during the anesthetic procedure and product application.

The data collected included age, mechanism, burn characteristics, management and outcomes. The hospitalization days, additional surgical intervention and all of the complications were recorded.

The children's characteristics were compared retrospectively with a control group, collected from the patients with the same type of injury who were treated with the standard of care (SoC). This group included the patients treated in the period before the implementation of enzymatic therapy in children in our center, or when Nexobrid® was unavailable.

The double assessment of burn wounds in the study group (before and after enzymatic debridement) was used to create a two-staged treatment algorithm.

An enzymatic debridement, such as the surgical removal of necrotic tissue, carries a risk of bleeding. The patients with bleeding disorders, such as bleeding diathesis, low platelet count, established anticoagulant therapy or an increased risk of active bleeding, are at a high risk of developing complications. A critical bleeding risk evaluation was performed on each child in the study and the SoC groups.

The study received approval from the Institutional Ethics Committee of the Independent Public District Hospital in Leczna (ref. number: 01/WCLO/2021).

The statistical analysis was carried out with Tibco Statistica 13.3 (StatSoft, Palo Alto, CA, USA). The values of the parameters were presented as arithmetic means and their standard deviations (SD) or number and percentage. The normal distribution of continuous variables was tested using the Shapiro–Wilk test. The continuous variables were analyzed using the test for parametric statistics for an intergroup comparison. The distributions of the discrete variables in groups were compared with the Pearson's chi-square test or Fisher's exact test. The relative risk (RR) and 95% confidence interval (using the approximation of Katz) were calculated. The error was set at 5% and significance at p-value < 0.05.

3. Results

3.1. Descriptive Analysis of the Study Group

A total of 12 children (6 females, 6 males; mean age 9 years, range 3 to 15 years) with mixed deep dermal and full thickness burn wounds were treated with Nexobrid®. None of the children had any significant comorbidities and were generally in good health, except for the burns. None were excluded from the study. The mean size of the burns was 29% (range 2–64%) total body surface area (TBSA), and all (100%) were mixed burns at presentation. The majority of the burns affected the upper extremities (83%), followed by the trunk (58%) and lower limbs (42%). The burns were caused by flame ($n = 6$), scalds ($n = 3$), hot oil ($n = 2$) or contact with a hot surface ($n = 1$). The patients were treated in different settings, depending on the age, depth of the burn, extension and location of the injury. A total of 6 out of 12 children had severe burns above 25% of TBSA and were treated in the intensive care unit. Three of them required temporary mechanical ventilation. The median percentage TBSA debrided using Nexobrid® was 15% (range 2–27%). In seven of the children, the enzymatic eschar removal of the entire burn surface was performed. In the remaining cases, some of the wounds qualified for conservative treatment, due to the high potential of spontaneous epithelialization in the primary assessment and the lack of a need for early surgical or enzymatic removal of necrotic tissue. The patient characteristics are summarized in Table 1.

Table 1. Characteristic of the study group treated enzymatically using Nexobrid® (NXB).

	Gender	Age	Cause	Depth	Total%	NXB %	Location of NXB	After NXB	STSG	Reconstruction	Length of Stay
1	M	12	flame	II/III	45%	9%	upper limbs	Skin grafts	yes (early)	no	38
2	F	5	flame	II/III	27%	27%	trunk, upper limbs	Skin grafts	yes (early)	z-plasty	77
3	F	3	scald	II/III	60%	20%	lower limbs	Suprathel	no	no	82
4	M	5	hot oil	II/III	39%	12%	trunk, lower limbs	Suprathel	yes (delayed)	z-plasty	33
5	F	3	scald	II/III	20%	20%	trunk, upper limbs	Suprathel	yes (delayed)	z-plasty	25
6	M	15	flame	II/III	2%	2%	upper limb	Jelonet + Gel	no	no	7
7	F	8	hot oil	II/III	7%	7%	trunk, upper limb	Jelonet + Gel	yes (delayed)	z-plasty	24
8	M	13	flame	II/III	47%	18%	trunk, limbs	Jelonet + Gel	yes (delayed)	z-plasty	37
9	F	10	flame	II/III	64%	25%	upper and lower limbs	Jelonet + Gel	yes (delayed)	z-plasty	28
10	M	12	flame	II/III	15%	15%	trunk, upper limb	skin grafts	yes (early)	no	29
11	M	9	scald	II/III	15%	15%	trunk, limbs	Suprathel	yes (delayed)	z-plasty	35
12	F	7	contact	II/III	7%	7%	upper limb	Mepithel	no	no	8

In a clinical assessment, the enzymatic debridement was effective in removing dead tissue in a single application in all twelve of the patients. Figures 1–4 show the enzymatic treatment in a 5-year-old child.

No adverse reaction to Nexobrid® was recorded in the study group. Early split thickness skin grafting (STSG) was used in three of the children, due to deep burns with no chance of spontaneous healing, as assessed after enzymatic debridement. The skin grafting was performed the day after the Nexobrid® application. In the other nine patients, various types of specialist dressings were used in the post enzymatic debridement wound care, to promote epithelialization. We used synthetic skin substitute (Suprathel®), paraffin tulle gras dressing (Jelonet®), wound gel with polyhexamethylene biguanide and betaine (Prontosan® Gel) and silicone net dressings (Mepithel®), in various configurations. In the period of 14–21 days after the injury, the wound epithelialization potential was assessed. In the patients with a lack of healing progress or in the event of pseudo-eschar, additional surgical procedures were applied. A total of six of nine children required additional debridement procedures and the covering of some of the wounds with STSG.

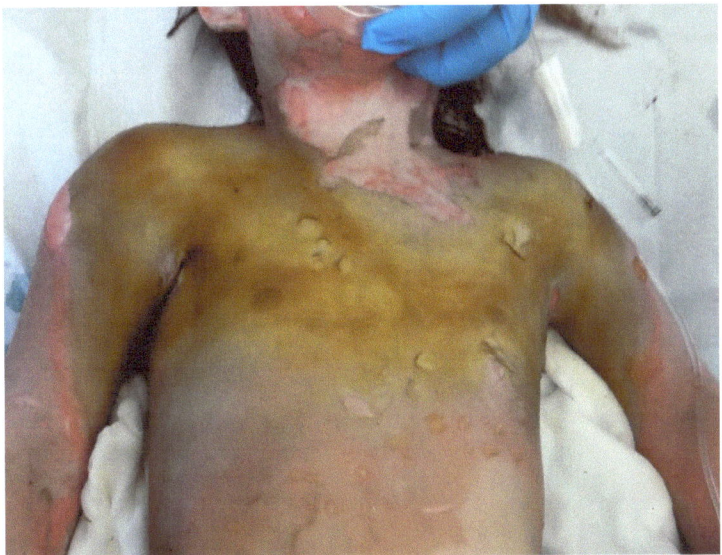

Figure 1. Burn on arrival.

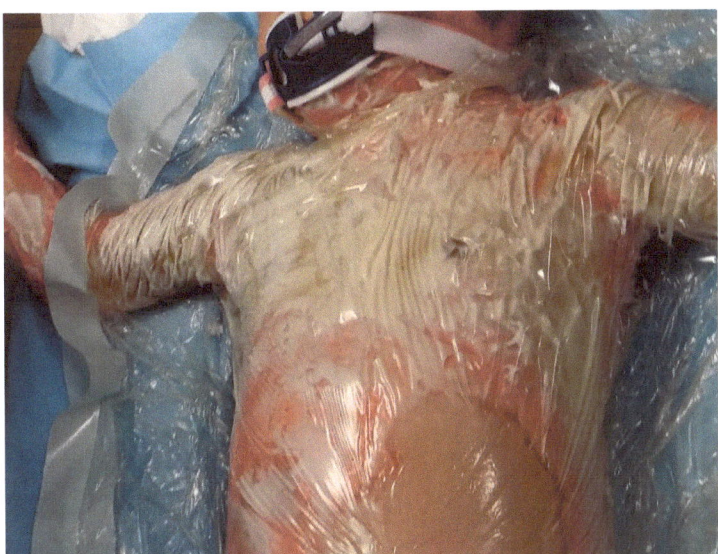

Figure 2. Nexobrid® application.

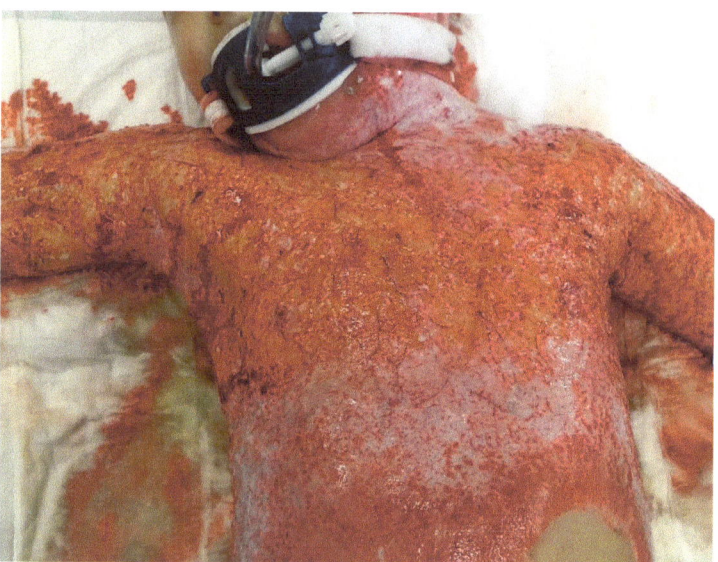

Figure 3. Result of enzymatic debridement.

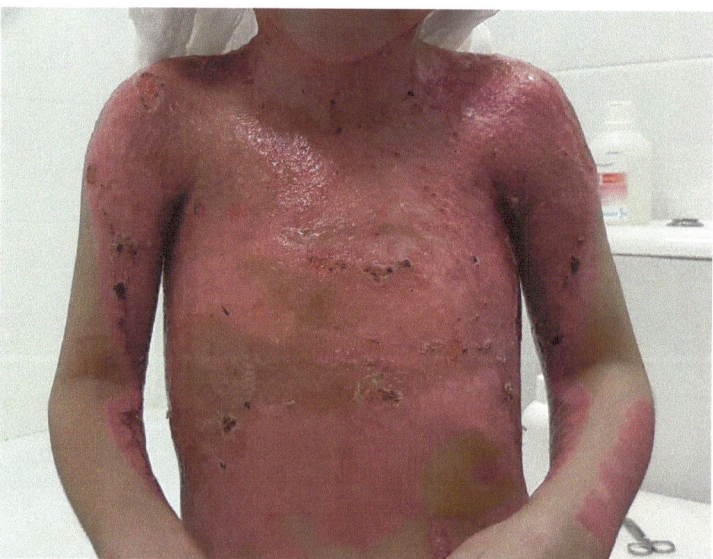

Figure 4. Final result (on discharge from hospital).

3.2. Comparison to SoC group

In the SoC group, 12 children (5 females, 7 males; mean age 9 years, range 2 to 17 years) with mixed deep dermal and full thickness burn wounds were treated with standard of care (SoC). Surgical necrectomy was performed in all of the children of this group (seven hydrosurgery using Versajet®, four tangential excision and one fascial excision). A total of 10 of the 12 children required skin grafts (five early and five delayed). In five patients, the surgically debrided wounds were simultaneously covered with STSG. The remaining five required additional debridement procedures and skin transplantation (STSG), due to the lack of spontaneous healing progress within 14–21 days after the injury.

The patient characteristics of SoC group are summarized in Table 2.

Table 2. Characteristic of the SoC group treated surgically.

	Gender	Age	Cause	Depth	Total%	Necrectomy%	Location of Necrectomy	Necrectomy	STSG	Reconstruction	Length of Stay
1	M	13	flame	II/III	57%	29%	trunk, limbs	fascial	yes (early)	ftsg	104
2	M	10	contact	II/III	4%	4%	trunk, upper limb	Versajet	yes (delayed)	no	21
3	M	7	flame	II/III	13%	10%	trunk, upper limb	Versajet	yes (delayed)	ftsg	28
4	M	3	flame	II/III	20%	10%	upper limbs	Versajet	yes (early)	z-plasty	39
5	F	4	scald	II/III	42%	15%	upper, lower limbs	tangential	yes (early)	matrix	78
6	M	17	flame	II/III	39%	18%	trunk, limbs	Versajet	yes (delayed)	z-plasty	36
7	M	8	scald	II/III	23%	5%	trunk, upper limbs	Versajet	yes (delayed)	ftsg	31
8	F	5	scald	II/III	7%	4%	upper limb	Versajet	no	no	27
9	M	13	flame	II/III	15%	15%	lower limbs	tangential	no	no	25
10	F	6	flame	II/III	74%	31%	head, trunk, limbs	Versajet	yes (early)	no	47
11	M	2	contact	II/III	2%	2%	upper limb	Versajet	yes (delayed)	matrix	44
12	F	15	flame	II/III	33%	24%	trunk, upper limbs	tangential	yes (early)	no	57

The study and the SoC groups were homogeneous in terms of age, type of injury, percentage of total burned area and percentage of debrided area. Wound colonization and infection rates did not differ in the pathogens identified on wound swabbing following enzymatic or surgical debridement. No significant bleeding complications were recorded in both of the groups. In the study group, hospitalization time varied from a minimum of 7 days to a maximum of 77 days, with an average of 35 days. The children in the comparison SoC group spent on average 27% more time in the hospital than the enzymatically treated patients. Although the hospitalization time of the study group is lower than that of the SoC group, the difference was not statistically significant ($p = 0.34$).

All of the children were discharged from the hospital with all of the wounds healed. In the 2-year follow-up period, two patients (17%) of the children treated with Nexobrid® required secondary reconstructive procedures due to burn contractures in the hand. In one case, Z-plasty was performed, in the other, the hypertrophic scar was removed following full thickness skin grafting (FTSG). In the SoC group, as many as seven children (58%) required the release of scar contractures (three FTSG, two Z-plasty and two skin matrix Nevelia®). The estimated relative risk of the need for secondary reconstructive procedures increased 3.5 times for the SoC group (RR 3.5, 95%CI 0.9–13.5, $p = 0.089$).

The comparison of results between study and SoC groups is presented in Table 3.

Table 3. Comparison of results between study and SoC groups.

	Total (n = 24)	Study Group (n = 12)	SoC Group (n = 12)	p-Value
Age (mean ± SD)	8.54 ± 4.38;	8.5 ± 4.01;	8.58 ± 4.96;	0.96
Gender (n, %)				
- male	14 (58.3)	6 (50.0)	8 (57.1)	0.68
- female	10 (41.7)	6 (50.0)	4 (33.3)	
Hospitalization (days) (mean ± SD)	40.0 ± 23.75;	35.25 ± 22.98;	44.75 ± 24.53;	0.34
Total burned area (%) (mean ± SD)	28 ± 21;	29 ± 21;	27 ± 22;	0.86
Debrided area (%) (mean ± SD)	14 ± 9;	15 ± 8;	14 ± 10;	0.82
Cause of a burn (n, %)				
flame	13 (54.2)	6 (50.0)	7 (58.3)	
scald	6 (25.0)	3 (25.0)	3 (25.0)	0.36
hot oil	2 (8.3)	2 (16.7)	0 (0)	
contact	3 (12.5)	1 (8.3)	2 (16.7)	
Skin grafting (STSG)				
early	8 (33.3)	3 (25.0)	5 (41.7)	0.79
delayed	11 (45.8)	6 (50.0)	5 (41.7)	
Reconstruction (n, %)	9 (37.5)	2 (16.7)	7 (58.3)	0.09

4. Discussion

Early eschar removal is the standard management of deep burns. The goal is to remove all of the necrotic tissue and render the wound suitable for healing or skin grafting [10,11]. The enzymatic debridement of burn wounds is an effective way to remove eschar [12]. Subsequently covering the wound with skin substitutes, specialist dressings or skin grafts, in turn, reduces the fluid loss and metabolic requirements, and protects the wound from the external environment. Thus, early debridement and proper wound management reduce the inflammation as well as preventing the risk of infection, wound sepsis and multiple organ failure [13,14].

The current European Medicines Agency license for enzymatic debridement using Nexobrid® limited its use to adults and to a maximum of 15% TBSA. The European and Polish Consensus, as well as the Italian recommendations, take into consideration enzymatic debridement for extensive burns but as an off-label use. Although, it is recommended to carry out enzymatic debridement in several stages, many of the centers in Europe had experience treating up to 25% TBSA in one session. The pretreatment risk stratification, adequate monitoring and hemodynamic support are needed when treating patients on more than 15% TBSA [15–17]. The literature lacks studies reporting the use of enzymatic debridement in children, with the exception of one manuscript presenting the combined experience in the use of Nexobrid® in pediatric burns throughout three clinical trials, and the study that explores the different possibilities for pain management during enzymatic debridement in pediatric and adult burn patients [18,19].

Since 2015, the Nexobrid® was added to the set of debridement tools available to the surgeon in our burn center. We gained significant knowledge during that time, starting with minor deep burns in adults. The studies confirming the safety of enzymatic debridement, as well as our experience in using this method, allowed us to extend the use of Nexobrid® on larger areas and on burn wounds in children [20,21]. One of the most important advantages of enzymatic debridement using Nexobrid® is its selective action. It removes eschar, leaving behind viable tissue [22,23]. The group of pediatric patients presented in this study was characterized by mixed deep dermal and full thickness burns. In this cases, it is difficult to clearly and precisely differentiate the depth, and thus the potential for spontaneous healing, or to make a decision for surgical excision and skin transplantation. Here, the enzymatic debridement appears to be the method of choice [24].

Enzymatic debridement is an effective diagnostic tool by assessing the wound after eschar removal, including bleeding patterns. It allows for the choice of an even better treatment strategy [25,26]. In our series, a total of only three patients underwent early autografting after Nexobrid® use, compared to five patients in the control group. In most of the cases, the primary burn assessment defined wounds as deep, qualified for early surgical excision and grafting. However, after enzymatic debridement, we observed the vital layers with the dermal architecture remaining upon removal of the enzyme, which impacted on our wound management. We could apply conservative treatment, achieve spontaneous healing in some areas and reduce the need for skin transplants. Therefore, we created an algorithm adapted to our demands including a double assessment of the burn wound before and after enzymatic debridement (Figure 5).

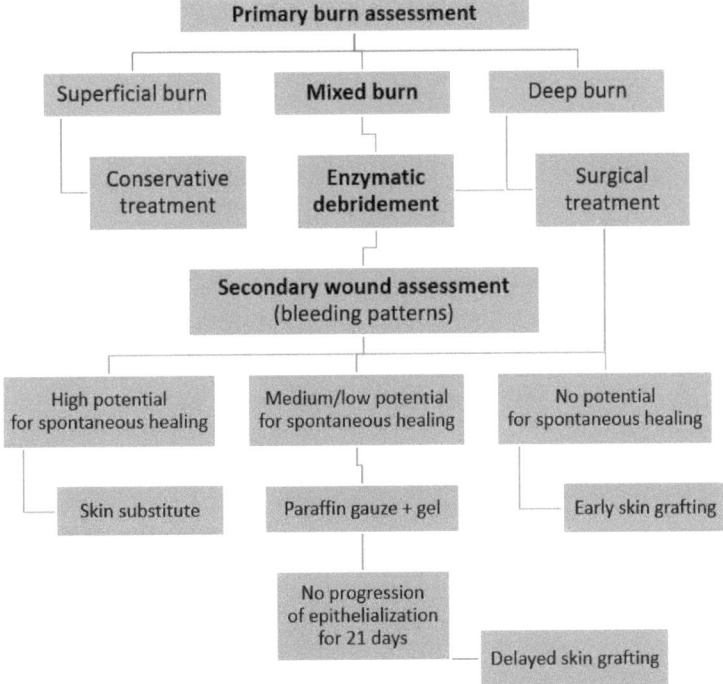

Figure 5. Treatment algorithm.

The presented strategy may have a positive effect on the number of additional surgical procedures and the duration of treatment. The children spent an average of 44.75 days inside the hospital in the SoC group, whereas only 35.25 days in the study group. The difference, however, is not statistically significant, which is in line with the results obtained by the Italian researchers on adults. They observed a reduced amount of autologous skin grafts, when the enzymatic method was applied, but the length of stay did not show significant differences compared to the surgically treated patients [27].

The early removal of the eschar with Nexobrid® is a safe and minimally invasive method. The enzymes are not harmful to healthy skin and preserve the vital dermis [21]. The study group had less skin grafts during the initial care compared to the SoC group. The number of reconstructive procedures due to scar contractures was reduced in the group treated enzymatically compared to the SoC-treated children. The children in the SoC group may have required more early skin grafting and reconstructive procedures because surgical excision is not as selective in salvaging areas of partial thickness in IIb/III burns as enzymatic debridement. Saving them from unnecessary surgery brings a significant benefit to patients and burn units. These results are in accordance with the results provided by a phase IIIb study of pediatric clinical trials. Autografting in deep partial thickness wounds was performed in 21.7% of the wounds debrided enzymatically vs. 31.8% of the wounds treated surgically ($p = 0.44$). The average long-term modified Vancouver Scar Scale scores were 3.4 for 18 wounds in 8 children treated with Nexobrid® versus 4.4 for 19 wounds in 9 children debrided using surgical methods [18]. Another study on adults showed a significant difference in the scar surface appearance (modified Yeong scale), with an average score of 2.5 in the study group, in comparison with 3.2 in SoC patients [27].

Most of the research focuses on Nexobrid® application to smaller areas, with particular emphasis on debriding burned hands [28–31]. Considering the safety and selectivity of this method, its use in children and severe burns seems even more justified. Recent publications addressing clinical off-label use of bromelain-based Nexobrid® in more excessive burns also confirm the usefulness of this method in the intensive care setting and during burn resuscitation [32,33]. Similarly, our study did not reveal any unexpected side effects or relevant adverse events after early enzymatic debridement, irrespective of the burn area.

The research presents some limitations. The data were collected retrospectively in a single-center and it should be emphasized that the population of children was small. Our study presents a preliminary report, rather than comprehensive data, and a small study population, however we hope it provides useful clinical guidance for other burn units wishing to use enzymatic debridement in severely burned children. Future extended, comparative or randomized trials are needed to confirm our results.

5. Conclusion

The enzymatic debridement using Nexobrid® is one of the effective methods of removing burn eschar in children, which the burn unit has at its disposal. The majority of thermal burns in children are of mixed depth, and Nexobrid® has an advantage over traditional necrectomy procedures due to its selectivity in identifying the areas of partial thickness burns and preserving these areas from unnecessary skin grafting, that could improve the patient outcomes and reduce hospital costs. The two-staged treatment-algorithm presented in this study became particularly useful, in order to avoid the need for secondary surgery. The main outcome of interest was the number of reconstructive procedures due to scar contractures, which was reduced in the group that was treated enzymatically compared to the SoC-treated children.

The experience of our burn center with the Bromelain-based eschar removal in children and in high % of TBSA suggests that this method offers a good and safe option to improve the treatment and life quality of children with severe burns.

Author Contributions: Conceptualization, T.K., E.G., J.S. and K.T.; methodology, T.K., E.G., J.S., M.B.-T., A.S., I.K.-G., M.S. and K.T.; software, T.K., E.G., J.S., M.B.-T., A.S., I.K.-G., M.S. and K.T.; validation, T.K., E.G., J.S., M.B.-T., A.S., I.K.-G., M.S. and K.T.; formal analysis, T.K., E.G., J.S., M.B.-T., A.S., M.S. and K.T.; investigation, T.K., E.G., J.S., M.B.-T., A.S., I.K.-G. and K.T.; resources T.K., E.G., J.S., M.B.-T., A.S., M.S. and K.T.; data curation, T.K., E.G., J.S., M.B.-T., A.S., M.S. and K.T.; writing—original draft preparation, T.K., E.G., J.S., M.B.-T., A.S., M.S. and K.T.; writing—review and editing, T.K., E.G., M.S. and K.T.; visualization, T.K., E.G., J.S., M.B.-T., A.S., I.K.-G., M.S. and K.T.; supervision, T.K., E.G. and K.T.; project administration, T.K., E.G., J.S., M.B.-T., A.S., M.S. and K.T.; funding acquisition, K.T. All authors have read and agreed to the published version of the manuscript.

Funding: This research was funded by the Medical University of Lublin, grants no. DS495 and no. GI10.

Institutional Review Board Statement: The study was conducted in accordance with the Declaration of Helsinki, and approved by the Institutional Ethics Committee of the Independent Public District Hospital in Leczna (ref. number: 01/WCLO/2021).

Informed Consent Statement: Informed consent was obtained from all subjects involved in the study.

Data Availability Statement: Not applicable.

Conflicts of Interest: The authors declare no conflict of interest.

References

1. Xiao-Wu, W.; Herndon, D.N.; Spies, M.; Sanford, A.P.; Wolf, S.E. Effects of delayed wound excision and grafting in severely burned children. *Arch. Surg.* **2002**, *137*, 1049–1054. [CrossRef] [PubMed]
2. Pruitt, B.A., Jr.; McManus, A.T.; Kim, S.H.; Goodwin, C.W. Burn wound infections: Current status. *World J. Surg.* **1998**, *22*, 135–145.
3. Williams, F.N.; Lee, J.O. Pediatric burn infection. *Surg. Infect. (Larchmt)* **2021**, *22*, 54–57. [CrossRef] [PubMed]
4. Daugherty, T.H.F.; Ross, A.; Neumeister, M.W. Surgical Excision of Burn Wounds. *Clin. Plast. Surg.* **2017**, *44*, 619–625. [CrossRef] [PubMed]
5. Tompkins, R.G.; Remensnyder, J.P.; Burke, J.F.; Tompkins, D.M.; Hilton, J.F.; Schoenfeld, D.A.; Behringer, G.E.; Bondoc, C.C.; Briggs, S.E.; Quinby, W.C., Jr. Significant reductions in mortality for children with burn injuries through the use of prompt eschar excision. *Ann. Surg.* **1988**, *208*, 577–585. [CrossRef] [PubMed]
6. Barret, J.P.; Herndon, D.N. Effects of burn wound excision on bacterial colonization and invasion. *Plast. Reconstr. Surg.* **2003**, *111*, 744–750. [CrossRef]
7. Griffin, B.; Bairagi, A.; Jones, L.; Dettrick, Z.; Holbert, M.; Kimble, R. Early non-excisional debridement of paediatric burns under general anaesthesia reduces time to re-epithelialisation and risk of skin graft. *Sci. Rep.* **2021**, *11*, 23753. [CrossRef]
8. Rosenberg, L.; Krieger, Y.; Bogdanov-Berezovski, A.; Silberstein, E.; Shoham, Y.; Singer, A.J. A novel rapid and selective enzymatic debridement agent for burn wound management: A multi-center RCT. *Burns* **2014**, *40*, 466–474. [CrossRef]
9. Loo, Y.L.; Goh, B.K.L.; Jeffery, S. An Overview of the Use of Bromelain-Based Enzymatic Debridement (Nexobrid®) in Deep Partial and Full Thickness Burns: Appraising the Evidence. *J. Burn Care Res.* **2018**, *39*, 932–938. [CrossRef]
10. Janzekovic, Z. A new concept in the early excision and immediate grafting of burns. *J. Trauma.* **1970**, *10*, 1103–1108. [CrossRef]
11. Orgill, D.P. Excision and skin grafting of thermal burns. *N. Engl. J. Med.* **2009**, *360*, 893–901. [CrossRef] [PubMed]
12. Hirche, C.; Citterio, A.; Hoeksema, H.; Koller, J.; Lehner, M.; Martinez, J.R.; Monstrey, S.; Murray, A.; Plock, J.A.; Sander, F.; et al. Eschar removal by bromelain based enzymatic debridement (Nexobrid®) in burns: An European consensus. *Burns* **2017**, *43*, 1640–1653. [CrossRef] [PubMed]
13. Ong, Y.S.; Samuel, M.; Song, C. Meta-Analysis of early excision of burns. *Burns* **2006**, *32*, 145–150. [CrossRef] [PubMed]
14. Saaiq, M.; Zaib, S.; Ahmad, S. Early excision and grafting versus delayed excision and grafting of deep thermal burns up to 40% total body surface area: A comparison of outcome. *Ann. Burn. Fire Disasters* **2012**, *25*, 143–147.
15. Hirche, C.; Almeland, S.K.; Dheansa, B.; Fuchs, P.; Governa, M.; Hoeksema, H.; Korzeniowski, T.; Lumenta, D.B.; Marinescu, S.; Martinez-Mendez, J.R.; et al. Eschar removal by bromelain based enzymatic debridement (Nexobrid®) in burns: European consensus guidelines update. *Burns* **2020**, *46*, 782–796. [CrossRef]
16. Ranno, R.; Vestita, M.; Maggio, G.; Verrienti, P.; Melandri, D.; Orlandi, C.; Perniciaro, G.; De Angelis, A.; D'Alessio, R.; Mataro, I.; et al. Italian recommendations on enzymatic debridement in burn surgery. *Burns* **2021**, *47*, 408–416. [CrossRef]
17. Korzeniowski, T.; Strużyna, J.; Chrapusta, A.M.; Krajewski, A.; Kucharzewski, M.; Piorun, K.; Nowakowski, J.; Surowiecka, A.; Kozicka, M.; Torres, K. A Questionnaire-Based Study to Obtain a Consensus from 5 Polish Burns Centers on Eschar Removal by Bromelain-Based Enzymatic Debridement (Nexobrid®) in Burns Following the 2020 Updated European Consensus Guidelines. *Med. Sci. Monit.* **2022**, *28*, e935632. [CrossRef]
18. Shoham, Y.; Krieger, Y.; Rubin, G.; Koenigs, I.; Hartmann, B.; Sander, F.; Schulz, A.; David, K.; Rosenberg, L.; Silberstein, E. Rapid enzymatic burn debridement: A review of the paediatric clinical trial experience. *Int. Wound J.* **2020**, *17*, 1337–1345. [CrossRef]
19. Claes, K.E.Y.; Amar, S.; Hoeksema, H.; Kornhaber, R.; de Jong, A.; Monstrey, S.; Haik, J.; Biros, E.; Harats, M. Pain management during a bromelain-based selective enzymatic debridement in paediatric and adult burn patients. *Burns* **2021**, *5*, 555–567. [CrossRef]
20. Rosenberg, L.; Lapid, O.; Bogdanov-Berezovsky, A.; Glesinger, R.; Krieger, Y.; Silberstein, E.; Sagi, A.; Judkins, K.; Singer, A.J. Safety and efficacy of a proteolytic enzyme for enzymatic burn debridement: A preliminary report. *Burns* **2004**, *30*, 843–850. [CrossRef]
21. Rosenberg, L.; Shoham, Y.; Krieger, Y.; Rubin, G.; Sander, F.; Koller, J.; David, K.; Egosi, D.; Ahuja, R.; Singer, A.J. Minimally invasive burn care: A review of seven clinical studies of rapid and selective debridement using a bromelain-based debriding enzyme (Nexobrid®). *Ann. Burn. Fire Disasters* **2015**, *28*, 264–274.
22. Schulz, A.; Fuchs, P.C.; Rothermundt, I.; Hoffmann, A.; Rosenberg, L.; Shoham, Y.; Oberländer, H.; Schiefer, J. Enzymatic debridement of deeply burned faces: Healing and early scarring based on tissue preservation compared to traditional surgical debridement. *Burns* **2017**, *43*, 1233–1243. [CrossRef] [PubMed]
23. Schulz, A.; Shoham, Y.; Rosenberg, L.; Rothermund, I.; Perbix, W.; Christian Fuchs, P.; Lipensky, A.; Schiefer, J.L. Enzymatic versus traditional surgical debridement of severely burned hands: A comparison of selectivity, efficacy, healing time, and threemonth scar quality. *J. Burn Care Res.* **2017**, *38*, e745–e755. [CrossRef] [PubMed]
24. Krieger, Y.; Bogdanov-Berezovsky, A.; Gurfinkel, R.; Silberstein, E.; Sagi, A.; Rosenberg, L. Efficacy of enzymatic debridement of deeply burned hands. *Burns* **2012**, *38*, 108–112. [CrossRef]

25. Schulz, A.; Perbix, W.; Shoham, Y.; Daali, S.; Charalampaki, C.; Fuchs, P.C.; Schiefer, J. Our initial learning curve in the enzymatic debridement of severely burned hands-Management and pit falls of initial treatments and our development of a post debridement wound treatment algorithm. *Burns* **2017**, *43*, 326–336. [CrossRef]
26. Krieger, Y.; Rubin, G.; Schulz, A.; Rosenberg, N.; Levi, A.; Singer, A.J.; Rosenberg, L.; Shoham, Y. Bromelain-based enzymatic debridement and minimal invasive modality (mim) care of deeply burned hands. *Ann. Burn. Fire Disasters* **2017**, *30*, 198–204.
27. Bernagozzi, F.; Orlandi, C.; Purpura, V.; Morselli, P.G.; Melandri, D. The Enzymatic Debridement for the Treatment of Burns of Indeterminate Depth. *J. Burn Care Res.* **2020**, *41*, 1084–1091. [CrossRef]
28. Dadras, M.; Wagner, J.M.; Wallner, C.; Sogorski, A.; Sacher, M.; Harati, K.; Lehnhardt, M.; Behr, B. Enzymatic debridement of hands with deep burns: A single center experience in the treatment of 52 hands. *J. Plast. Surg. Hand Surg.* **2020**, *54*, 220–224. [CrossRef]
29. Corrales-Benítez, C.; González-Peinado, D.; González-Miranda, Á.; Martínez-Méndez, J.R. Evaluation of burned hand function after enzymatic debridement. *J. Plast. Reconstr. Aesthet. Surg.* **2021**, *22*, 1048–1056. [CrossRef]
30. Ziegler, B.; Hundeshagen, G.; Cordts, T.; Kneser, U.; Hirche, C. State of the art in enzymatic debridement. *Plast. Aesthet. Res.* **2018**, *5*, 33. [CrossRef]
31. Siegwart, L.C.; Böcker, A.H.; Diehm, Y.F.; Kotsougiani-Fischer, D.; Erdmann, S.; Ziegler, B.; Kneser, U.; Hirche, C.; Fischer, S. Enzymatic Debridement for Burn Wound Care: Interrater Reliability and Impact of Experience in Post-intervention Therapy Decision. *J. Burn Care Res.* **2021**, *42*, 953–961. [CrossRef] [PubMed]
32. Hofmaenner, D.A.; Steiger, P.; Schuepbach, R.A.; Klinzing, S.; Waldner, M.; Klein, H.; Enthofer, K.; Giovanoli, P.; Mannil, L.; Buehler, P.K.; et al. Safety of enzymatic debridement in extensive burns larger than 15% total body surface area. *Burns* **2021**, *47*, 796–804. [CrossRef] [PubMed]
33. Bowers, C.; Randawa, A.; Sloan, B.; Anwar, U.; Phipps, A.; Muthayya, P. Enzymatic debridement in critically injured burn patients—Our experience in the intensive care setting and during burn resuscitation. *Burns* **2021**, *12*, 846–859. [CrossRef] [PubMed]

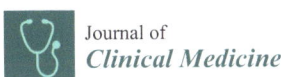

Article

Three Different Types of Fat Grafting for Facial Systemic Sclerosis: A Case Series

Antonio Arena [1], Umberto Committeri [1], Fabio Maglitto [1], Giovanni Salzano [2,*], Giovanni Dell'Aversana Orabona [1], Luigi Angelo Vaira [3], Pasquale Piombino [1], Michela Apolito [1], Gianluca Renato De Fazio [1] and Luigi Califano [1]

[1] Maxillofacial Surgery Operative Unit, Department of Neurosciences, Reproductive and Odontostomatological Sciences, Federico II University of Naples, 80131 Naples, Italy
[2] Division of Surgical Oncology Maxillo-Facial Unit, Istituto Nazionale Tumori-IRCCS-Fondazione G. Pascale, Via Mariano Semmola, 80131 Naples, Italy
[3] Maxillofacial Surgery Operative Unit, University Hospital of Sassari, 07100 Sassari, Italy
* Correspondence: giovanni.salzano@istitutotumori.na.it

Citation: Arena, A.; Committeri, U.; Maglitto, F.; Salzano, G.; Dell'Aversana Orabona, G.; Vaira, L.A.; Piombino, P.; Apolito, M.; De Fazio, G.R.; Califano, L. Three Different Types of Fat Grafting for Facial Systemic Sclerosis: A Case Series. *J. Clin. Med.* **2022**, *11*, 5489. https://doi.org/10.3390/jcm11185489

Academic Editor: Mieszko Wieckiewicz

Received: 2 August 2022
Accepted: 15 September 2022
Published: 19 September 2022

Publisher's Note: MDPI stays neutral with regard to jurisdictional claims in published maps and institutional affiliations.

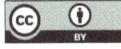

Copyright: © 2022 by the authors. Licensee MDPI, Basel, Switzerland. This article is an open access article distributed under the terms and conditions of the Creative Commons Attribution (CC BY) license (https:// creativecommons.org/licenses/by/ 4.0/).

Abstract: Systemic sclerosis (SSc) is a heterogeneous, chronic connective tissue disease, characterized by skin fibrosis as well as vascular and visceral lesions. It can involve the lungs, heart, kidneys, gastrointestinal tract, and bones. The orofacial manifestations of SSc can cause functional, aesthetic, and social distress, resulting in significant psychological implications for the patients. In recent decades, fat grafting improved the aesthetic outcomes in terms of volume deficiency, contour asymmetry, and skin elasticity of the face thanks to the regenerative action of the stem cells contained within it. We describe five cases of a patient with SSc treated with fat grafting used to correct volume loss and facial elasticity of the lips and perioral region on the middle and lower third of the face. All the patients received regular postoperative checks at weeks 1 and 2. A multiple choice questionnaire was administered to assess the degree of tolerability of the procedure. The reliability of the questionnaire was evaluated by calculating the Cronbach alpha using the MedCalc Statistical Software version 20.113. The aim of our study is to describe three different types of fat grafting used to correct volume loss and restore facial elasticity of the lips and perioral region on the middle and lower third of the face.

Keywords: systemic sclerosis; fat graft; orofacial SSc; maxillo-facial surgery; lipofilling

1. Introduction

Systemic sclerosis (SSc) is a heterogeneous, chronic connective tissue disease, characterized by skin fibrosis and vascular and visceral lesions. It involves the lungs, heart, kidneys, gastrointestinal tract, and bones [1].

Two subtypes with cutaneous involvement have been described: limited cutaneous SSc and diffuse cutaneous SSc. In both of them, the face is frequently affected, with related aesthetic and functional disorders [2,3].

Due to the loss of elasticity and skin fibrosis, the face's involvement in SSc often causes a "mask appearance" and microstomy, compromising some regular daily activities, such as eating, talking, drinking, and practicing regular oral hygiene.

The orofacial manifestations of SSc can cause functional, aesthetic, and social distress, resulting in significant psychological implications for the patients.

As reported in the literature, in recent decades, fat grafting improved the aesthetic outcomes in terms of volume deficiency, contour asymmetry, and skin elasticity of the face, thanks to the regenerative action of the stem cells contained within it.

The aim of our study is to describe three different types of fat grafting used to correct volume loss and facial elasticity of the lips and perioral region on the middle and lower third of the face.

2. Materials and Methods

Five consecutive patients underwent fat grafting for SSc with aspects of diffuse cutaneous sclerosis between January 2021 and June 2021 at the Maxillo-Facial Surgery Unit of the University of Naples "Federico II". All the patients were informed about the procedure and signed a preoperative consent for data recording in our clinical database. All patients underwent clinical facial analysis before the procedure. The patients presented the typical mask-like appearance of the face, with hypotrophy of the middle and lower third, labial incompetence with microstomy, and limited mouth opening. Hypoelasticity and thickening of the skin was highlighted, especially in the perioral and labial region. All of them mostly complained about difficulties in daily activities, such as talking, drinking, or eating, with frequent drooling, fatigue, and considerable psychological distress.

For these reasons, we decided to improve skin elasticity and volume loss through three different type of fat grafting. This study was approved by the Federico II University Ethics Committee (protocol N.81/20) on 2 April 2020.

2.1. Surgical Technique

The procedure was performed under general anesthesia, and the abdomen was the donor site. A modified Klein solution composed of 1 Lt saline solution with 100 mL of 1% plain lidocaine and 1 ml of 1:1000 adrenaline was injected into the donor site through a 14-gauge spiral, multi-port tumescent infiltrator cannula (Tulip Medical, San Diego, CA, USA) to obtain hydro-dissection and fat tumescence. An atraumatic liposuction using a 14 G × 15 cm Carraway Harvester with a spiral three-port design (Tulip Medical, San Diego, CA, USA) on a 20 mL luer-lock syringe with a low suction pressure allowed us to collect 90 cc of raw adipose tissue. The fat obtained was washed several times with a saline solution, and a gravity separation was achieved.

Three different modalities to process the harvested fat were performed (Figure 1):

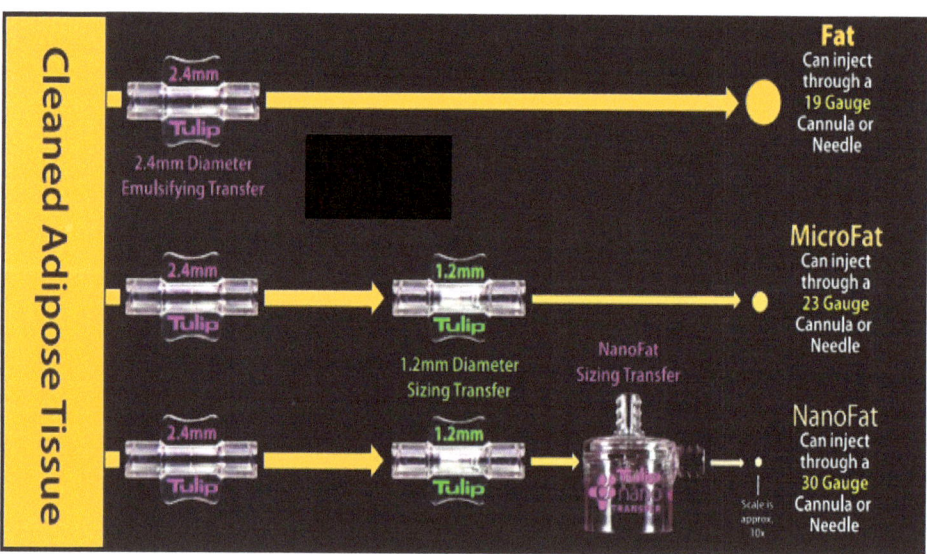

Figure 1. Harvested fat processing procedure sequence.

Macrofat: 20 cc of fat obtained was transferred in a 3 cc luer-lock syringe through a Luer to Luer 2.4 mm Anaerobic Transfer (Tulip Medical, San Diego, CA, USA).

Microfat: 15 cc of fat obtained was processed by an intersyringe shuffle using a Luer to Luer 2.4 mm Anaerobic Transfer (Tulip Medical, San Diego, CA, USA). After 20 passes, the same process was repeated through Luer-Lock 1.2 mm Connector (Tulip Medical, San Diego, CA, USA) for the other 15 passes.

Nanofat: the same two steps applied to obtain the microfat were performed starting from 20 cc of harvested fat. Using a 400-micron filter NanoTransfer (Tulip Medical, San Diego, CA, USA), the connective tissue remnants were removed.

Macrofat was used to restore the volume of the lip, perioral rim, and zygomatic area after a skin and dermis penetration with an 18-gauge needle in four entry points. The entry points were symmetrical for both facial sides and were positioned 1 cm laterally in the labial commissure and in the area between the midcheek and the zygomatic arch (Figures 2 and 3).

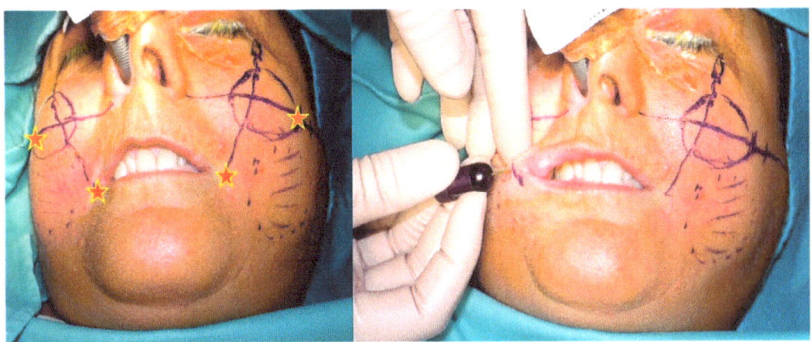

Figure 2. Surgical marking and entry points (indicated as pentagrams) of procedure.

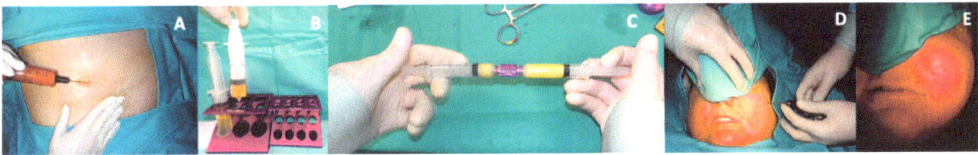

Figure 3. Fat collection from the abdominal region (**A**), fat decanting (**B**), fat processing (**C**), fat grafting (**D**), and the immediate postoperative state (**E**).

Approximately 3.5 to 5 mL of fat per side was injected with a single orifice 18-gauge × 7 cm microinjector cannula (Tulip Medical, San Diego, CA, USA). The quantity of fat injected was based on the morphology of the patient's face. Microfat was placed to improve the nasolabial folds and the cheekbone area through the same entry points used for the macrofat. An amount of 1.5 to 2.5 mL of fat per side was injected with a retrograde fan technique using a 20-gauge × 5 cm single orifice blunt cannula (Tulip Medical, San Diego, CA, USA). Nanofat was injected superficially in the perioral wrinkles and in the vermilion border using a 27-gauge needle. An amount of 2 to 3 mL of nanofat per side was injected using a retrograde linear technique.

2.2. Postprocedure Assessment

All the patients received regular postoperative specific checks at 1 and 2 weeks as well as at 6 months and 1 year after the procedure (Figure 4). A multiple choice questionnaire was administered to assess the degree of tolerability of the procedure and the aesthetic and functional outcomes. A postoperative evaluation of pain and itching was requested 2 weeks after surgery; aesthetic and functional improvements were evaluated at the 6-month check.

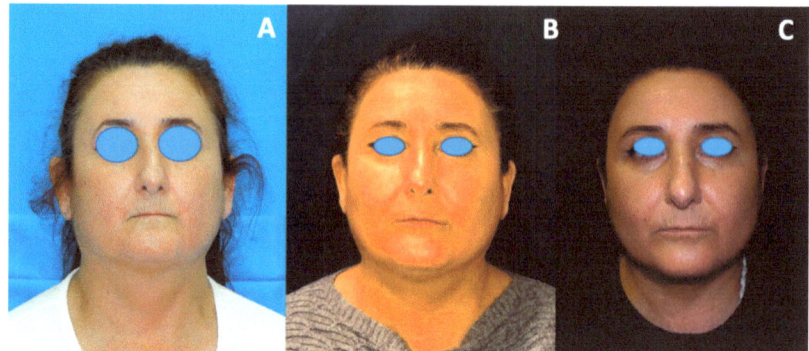

Figure 4. Preoperative (**A**), 6 months postoperative (**B**), 1 year postoperative (**C**).

The questionnaire was built and evaluated according to a 5-point Likert scale. The five items included the following:

1. Pain;
2. Itching;
3. Tissue elasticity;
4. Degree of aesthetic satisfaction;
5. Lip competence.

For each question, the patient could give a score from 1 up to 5 corresponding to the degree of tolerability. A score ranging from 20 to 25 was considered very good, from 15 to 19 was considered good, from 10 to 14 was considered acceptable, and <9 was considered poor. The reliability of the questionnaire was evaluated by calculating the Cronbach alpha using the software MedCalc Statistical Software version 20.113 (MedCalc Software bv, Ostend, Belgium; https://www.medcalc.org; accessed on 16 October 2020).

3. Results

In our sample, there were 5 patients (3F, 2M). No surgical complications were detected during outpatients' checks. No other complications, such as allergic reactions or hematoma directly related with the procedure, were reported.

The reliability of the administered questionnaire was confirmed by the Cronbach alpha being equal to 0.83 with raw variables and 0.85 with standardized variables. The effect of the mask on the 5 items defined in the administered questionnaire is reported in Figure 5. The overall results are reported in Table 1. Three patients reported a very good result, giving a score between 20 and 25 (mean 20.67), and two patients reported a good result, giving a score between 15 and 19 (mean 18). The total average score was 19.6.

Table 1. Patients' questionnaire answers.

	Q1	Q2	Q3	Q4	Q5
Pz 1	4	5	5	3	4
Pz 2	4	3	4	3	4
Pz 3	3	3	4	5	5
Pz 4	5	4	5	3	4
Pz 5	3	3	3	5	4

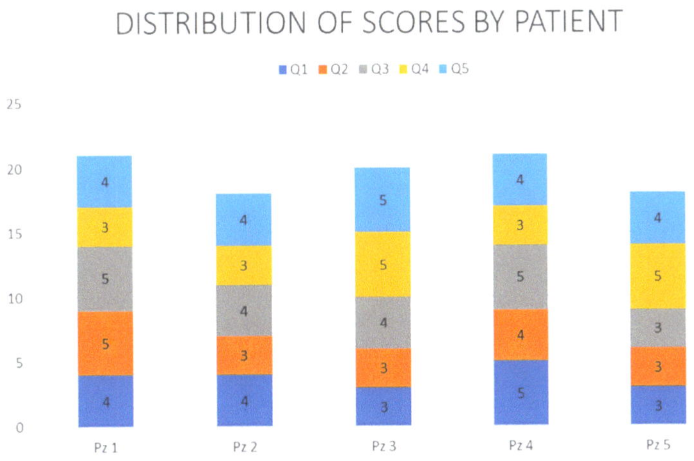

DISTRIBUTION OF SCORES BY PATIENT

■ Q1 ■ Q2 ■ Q3 ■ Q4 ■ Q5

Patient	Q1	Q2	Q3	Q4	Q5
Pz 1	4	5	5	3	4
Pz 2	4	3	4	3	4
Pz 3	3	4	5	3	5
Pz 4	5	4	3	3	4
Pz 5	3	3	3	5	4

Figure 5. Distribution of score.

4. Discussion

SSc is a chronic autoimmune disease of unknown etiology, characterized by diffuse fibrosis, abnormal immune system activation, and skin, joint, and internal organ microvascular anomalies. In particular, the complications of the internal organs are the main causes of the high mortality rate. It is more common among women, especially between the ages of 20 and 50.

This disease is highly disabling for the patient due to the aesthetic and functional outcomes that limit daily life. The most frequent symptoms include Raynaud's phenomenon, polyarthralgia, dysphagia, heartburn, swelling, and, eventually, retraction of the fingers and skin fibrosis. [1] Skin and visceral organ fibrosis is caused by the synthesis and deposition of the extracellular matrix and collagen determined by profibrotic myofibroblasts [4–6].

SSc can be divided into limited systemic sclerosis, formerly referred to as CREST syndrome (calcinosis of the skin, Raynaud's phenomenon, esophageal motility disorders, sclerodactyly, telangiectasia); generalized systemic sclerosis (with widespread skin involvement); systemic sclerosis without scleroderma; and overlap syndromes that present the typical symptoms of other connectivitis.

The most evident feature of the full-blown disease is the presence of skin fibrosis, as indicated by the name scleroderma.

In the initial forms, it occurs only with edema. In advanced forms, the disease is characterized by loss of skin elasticity, smoothing of expression lines on the face, difficulty opening the oral rim, lip resorption (microcheilia), and difficulty completely moving the joints, especially the hands that tend to assume a curved ("claw") attitude with hindrances in the extension and fine movements of the fingers.

Recently, the use of autologous fat grafting in SSc has allowed a reduction of the effects of skin fibrosis caused by the disease. As reported in the literature, fat grafting has already been used in various conditions such as scars, post-traumatic deformities, radiodermatitis, congenital anomalies, contour abnormalities, burn injuries, breast capsular contracture and augmentation, cosmetic procedures, and also localized forms of scleroderma such as "en coup de saber" [7–10]. As described for the first time by Coleman, we used the lipofilling technique on our patient, which consisted of taking a fat graft from a donor site (abdomen, thigh, buttock) to a recipient one [11]. Based on the technique of extraction and manipulation of the harvested tissue, we obtained three different types by size: macrofat graft for the subcutaneous tissue, microfat graft for the deep dermis, and nanofat graft for the superficial dermis.

In particular, the macrofat was infiltrated for its volumizing effect. Microfat has been exploited for its regenerative and filling action in the cheekbone, lip, and nasolabial fold region [12]. The biorevitalizing effect of nanofat improved perioral wrinkles and the motility of the lips, increasing the mouth opening. During the procedure, cannulas and needles of different sizes were used in the different facial areas due to the type of injection.

In addition to its filling effect, the high number of mesenchymal stem cells (ASCs) obtained with this technique represent the major advantage compared to any other body tissue graft [13]. The regenerative power of ASCs is attributable to their ability to secrete angiogenic factors and immunomodulatory properties that facilitate tissue repair [14,15].

The limit of the procedure is represented by the survival time of the grafted fat and by the long follow-up, both due in part to the reabsorption of the adipose tissue and to the long times of differentiation of the stem cells and of the angiogenic processes [16].

5. Conclusions

In conclusion, this surgical technique resulted in a greater elasticity of the skin tissue, a smoothing of the perioral wrinkles, and an improvement in microstomy, drooling, and fatigue. On the other hand, no effect was found on the increase in the volume of the zygomatic region and the lips, probably due to the reduced follow-up and partial reabsorption of the tissue.

To achieve the ideal volume and more evident results, which can improve the quality of life in carrying out daily activities, repeated injections are indicated [17,18].

Author Contributions: Conceptualization, A.A. and F.M.; methodology, U.C.; validation, L.A.V. and P.P.; formal analysis, G.D.O.; investigation, G.S.; resources, M.A.; data curation, G.R.D.F.; writing—original draft preparation, A.A. and U.C.; writing—review and editing, F.M.; visualization, G.R.D.F.; supervision, G.D.O.; project administration, L.C. All authors have read and agreed to the published version of the manuscript.

Funding: This research received no external funding.

Institutional Review Board Statement: The study was conducted in accordance with the Declaration of Helsinki.

Informed Consent Statement: Informed consent was obtained from all subjects involved in the study. Written informed consent has been obtained from the patient(s) to publish this paper.

Data Availability Statement: The data presented in this study are available on request from the corresponding author. The data are not publicly available due to privacy.

Conflicts of Interest: The authors declare no conflict of interest.

References

1. Hadj Said, M.; Foletti, J.M.; Graillon, N.; Guyot, L.; Chossegros, C. Orofacial manifestations of scleroderma. A literature review. *Rev. Stomatol. Chir. Maxillofac. Chir Orale.* **2016**, *117*, 322–326. [CrossRef] [PubMed]
2. Alhajeri, H.; Hudson, M.; Fritzler, M.; Pope, J.; Tatibouet, S.; Markland, J.; Robinson, D.; Jones, N.; Khalidi, N.; Docherty, P.; et al. 2013 American College of Rheumatology/European League against rheumatism classifcation criteria for systemic sclerosis outperform the 1980 criteria: Data from the Canadian Scleroderma Research Group. *Arthritis Care Res.* **2015**, *67*, 582–587. [CrossRef] [PubMed]
3. Panchbhai, S.; Pawar, A.B.; Kazi, Z. Review of orofacial considerations of systemic sclerosis or scleroderma with report of analysis of 3 cases. *Indian J. Dent.* **2016**, *7*, 134. [CrossRef] [PubMed]
4. Varga, J.; Trojanowska, M.; Kuwana, M. Pathogenesis of systemic sclerosis: Recent insights of molecular and cellular mechanisms and therapeutic opportunities. *J. Scleroderma Relat. Disord.* **2017**, *2*, 137–152. [CrossRef]
5. Denton, C.P.; Khanna, D. Systemic sclerosis. *Lancet* **2017**, *390*, 1685–1699. [CrossRef]
6. Abbate, V.; Dell'Aversana Orabona, G.; Seidita, F.; Committeri, U.; Bonavolontà, P.; Piombino, P.; Audino, G.; Iaconetta, G.; Califano, L. Facial Soft Tissue Ptosis: A Quantitative Analysis using 3d Facial Scan App For iPhone. *J. Maxillofac. Oral Surg.* **2022**. [CrossRef]

7. Bonavolontà, P.; Giovanni, D.O.; Goglia, F.; Romano, A.; Abbate, V.; Arena, A.; Iaconetta, G.; Califano, L. A new surgical approach for the treatment of Rhinophyma. *Ann. Ital. Chir.* **2020**, *9*, S2239253X20033150. [PubMed]
8. Clauser, L.C.; Tieghi, R.; Galiè, M.; Carinci, F. Structural fat grafting. *J. Craniofac. Surg.* **2011**, *22*, 1695–1701. [CrossRef] [PubMed]
9. Gir, P.; Brown, S.A.; Oni, G.; Kashefi, N.; Mojallal, A.; Rohrich, R.J. Fat grafting: Evidence-based review on autologous fat harvesting, processing, reinjection, and storage. *Plast. Reconstr. Surg.* **2012**, *130*, 249–258. [CrossRef] [PubMed]
10. Wetterau, M.; Szpalski, C.; Hazen, A.; Warren, S.M. Autologous fat grafting and facial reconstruction. *J. Craniofac. Surg.* **2012**, *23*, 315–318. [CrossRef] [PubMed]
11. Coleman, S.R. Structural fat grafting: More than a permanent filler. *Plast. Reconstr. Surg.* **2006**, *118*, 108S–120S. [CrossRef] [PubMed]
12. Sautereau, N.; Daumas, A.; Truillet, R.; Jouve, E.; Magalon, J.; Veran, J.; Casanova, D.; Frances, Y.; Magalon, G.; Granel, B. Efficacy of Autologous Microfat Graft on Facial Handicap in Systemic Sclerosis Patients. *Plast. Reconstr. Surg. Glob. Open* **2016**, *4*, e660. [CrossRef] [PubMed]
13. Bellini, E.; Grieco, M.P.; Raposio, E. The science behind autologous fat grafting. *Ann. Med. Surg.* **2017**, *24*, 65–73. [CrossRef] [PubMed]
14. Maglitto, F.; Sani, L.; Piloni, S.; Del Prete, G.D.; Arena, A.; Committeri, U.; Salzano, G.; Califano, L.; Friscia, M. Step-technique genioplasty: A case report. *Int. J. Surg. Case Rep.* **2022**, *95*, 107232. [CrossRef]
15. Magalon, G.; Daumas, A.; Sautereau, N.; Magalon, J.; Sabatier, F.; Granel, B. Regenerative Approach to Scleroderma with Fat Grafting. *Clin. Plast. Surg.* **2015**, *42*, 64–353. [CrossRef] [PubMed]
16. Pu, L.L.Q. Mechanisms of fat graft survival. *Ann. Plast. Surg.* **2016**, *77*, S84–S86. [CrossRef] [PubMed]
17. Friscia, M.; Bonavolontà, P.; Arena, A.; Committeri, U.; Maglitto, F.; Salzano, G.; Iaconetta, G.; Califano, L. Syngnathia: A rare case of maxillo-mandibular fusion in an adult patient. *Chirurgia* **2020**, *33*, 65–69. [CrossRef]
18. Ohashi, M. Fat Grafting for Facial Rejuvenation with Cryopreserved Fat Grafts. *Clin. Plast. Surg.* **2020**, *47*, 63–71. [CrossRef] [PubMed]

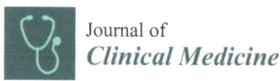

Article

Histopathological Evaluation of the Healing Process of Standardized Skin Burns in Rabbits: Assessment of a Natural Product with Honey and Essential Oils

Anis Anis [1,*], Ahmed Sharshar [2], Saber El Hanbally [3] and Awad A. Shehata [4,5,6,*]

1 Department of Pathology, Faculty of Veterinary Medicine, University of Sadat City, Sadat City 32958, Egypt
2 Department of Surgery, Anesthesiology and Radiology, Faculty of Veterinary Medicine, University of Sadat City, Sadat City 32958, Egypt
3 Department of Pharmacology, Faculty of Veterinary Medicine, University of Sadat City, Sadat City 32958, Egypt
4 Avian and Rabbit Diseases Department, Faculty of Veterinary Medicine, University of Sadat City, Sadat City 32958, Egypt
5 Research and Development Section, PerNaturam GmbH, 56290 Gödenroth, Germany
6 Prophy-Institute for Applied Prophylaxis, 59759 Bönen, Germany
* Correspondence: aniszaid@vet.usc.edu.eg (A.A.); awad.shehata@pernaturam.de (A.A.S.)

Abstract: Skin burns are one of the most difficult medical problems. Recently, studies have been directed towards development of natural products in order to identify effective and safe remedies. In the present study, we evaluated the efficacy of a natural composite (formulated from honey and essential oils) compared with MEBO® (0.25% β-sitosterol) and DERMAZIN® creams (1% silver-sulfadiazine) in the treatment of thermally induced skin burns. For this purpose, four burn-wounds were created on the back of male New Zealand rabbits ($n = 10$) using a thermal stamp under the effect of general anesthesia. Each wound represents one of the following groups: non-treated, natural composite-cream, MEBO®-cream, and silver-sulfadiazine treated groups, respectively. Treatments were applied once a day topically until one of these wounds appeared to be healed grossly. The non-treated group received no treatment. Grossly, skin burns have been healed after 28 days of the treatment in all groups except of the non-treated group. The healing efficacy of the natural composite, MEBO® and silver-sulfadiazine creams was quite similar macroscopically. However, microscopically, the epidermal layer of the composite-cream treated group was more mature than those of both MEBO® and silver-sulfadiazine creams treated groups. In conclusion, the tested composite may be a promising effective and inexpensive treatment of skin burns.

Keywords: regeneration; skin burns; natural; composite; rabbit; histopathology

1. Introduction

Burns are regarded as one of the most serious injuries. Physical impairments or even disabilities, as well as emotional and mental diseases, can result from burns. In developing countries, burns are one of the public health issues [1,2]. The World Health Organization (WHO) reported that each year approximately 11 million people suffer from burn wounds worldwide. About 180,000 of whom die because of such injuries and the non-fatal burn injuries are a leading cause of morbidity [3]. The majority of these cases occur in low- and middle-income countries in African and South-East Asia regions [3]. Additionally, skin burns are one of the complicated affections [4] which recorded in different animals [5–8]. However, to our knowledge, there is no documented data to measure the number of skin affections in animals, neither locally nor globally.

Burn injury can be classified according to its severity, depth, and size. Superficial burns (first-degree) are the type of burns that affect the uppermost layer of the skin (epidermis only), and skin becomes red with limited pain. Second-degree burns are divided into two types, superficial partial-thickness burns and deep partial-thickness burns. The superficial partial-thickness burns are characterized by painful, weep, and require dressing and wound care. However, the deep partial-thickness burns are less painful due to partial destruction of the pain receptors and require surgery. The third-degree burns affect the full thickness of the skin and are not typically painful due to the damage to the nerve endings and requires protection from becoming infected. Finally, the fourth-degree burns involve the underlying tissue such as muscle or bone and frequently accompanied by sloughing of burned tissues [9].

Skin burns can be induced by thermal, chemical, radioactive and electrical causes. Heat is one of the most common causes of skin burns which can induce a sudden coagulative necrosis of cells and tissues producing physical and physiological damage to the affected tissues resulting in enormous complications if not treated quickly and efficiently. Skin healing and regeneration of the complicated cases of skin burns need long hospitalization, expensive medications, and long rehabilitation programs [10–12].

Indeed, skin burns are quite common in animals, for example, dermal skin burns in pet animals has been reported after prolonged sun exposure especially in high ambient temperature as plaques and eschars. The microscopic features of theses lesions (like epidermal, vascular, and adnexal necrosis, and subepidermal vesiculation) were consistent with full-thickness thermal skin burns. The brown dachshund dogs are sensitive to direct sunlight exposure, which induce cutaneous skin burn [5,13,14]. Additionally, thermal skin burns have been recorded in small animals, most of these burns are caused by intentional or accidental exposure to a heat source, such as boiling liquids, electric heating pads, flames, hot air dryers, hot metals, and hot lamps [6]. Recently, other causes which induce skin injuries such as transdermal drug delivery has become a growing trend in veterinary medicine. Some substances that help in drug diffusion through the epidermis and subcutaneous tissues are known as penetration enhancers, sorption promoters, or accelerants. However, their uses in veterinary products with a high-absorbed dose may result in adverse side dermatological effects such as toxicological irritations [15].

Antibiotics are widely used in the treatment strategies of skin burns to prevent secondary infection, but unfortunately in some cases antibiotics may induce allergic reactions which delay the healing process [16]. Tissue engineered wound dressings and growth factors are also used in wound healing process but they are relatively too expensive. Therefore, studies for the discovery of new natural compounds that can be used in the healing process of skin burns are still required [10]. Several medicinal plants contain a vast diversity of phytogenic compound with antioxidant, anti-inflammatory and immunomodulatory properties [17] which can be the cornerstone of the future medication of burns.

Several natural products such as honey, rosemary and chamomile oils have many health benefits particularly in skin regeneration process. These natural bioactive substances were previously investigated individually as enhancers of wound healing [18–20]. In our previous study, combination between these materials enhanced the wound healing in equines [21]. Honey is one of the oldest known traditional treatments and it was declared in the Holy Quran since 1444 years ago. It has been employed for healing of several skin diseases including ulcers, wounds, eczema, and burns [22]. Honey has anti-inflammatory and antibacterial effects which decreasing edema and exudation. Additionally, honey stimulates tissue regeneration which promotes healing and diminishes the scar size [18].

Rosemary (*Rosmarinus officinalis* Linn.) is an aromatic plant which has therapeutic properties and has been used in pharmaceutical and cosmetics industries as well as in the folk medicine. Rosemary has antioxidant and anti-inflammatory properties due to the presence of carnosol/carnosic and ursolic acids. Rosemary has been used in the treatment of inflammatory diseases, wound healing, cancer, skin mycoses, cellulite, alopecia, ultraviolet damage, and aging [19,23–29]. Chamomile, family *Asteraceae*, is one of the most ancient herbal plants used in the herbal medicinal [30]. It contains several bioactive constituents [31]. Chamomile possesses antioxidant and anti-inflammatory properties in addition to its role in skin protection and regeneration of the necrosed skin [30–36]. Other oils of plant origin such as sesame oil [22,37,38] and olive oil [38,39] have been subjected to several experimental studies to evaluate their effects on the healing process of skin burns. Sesame oil is considered one of the most important sources of β-sitosterol which is one of the most powerful natural anti-inflammatory [7,40] which used to prevent and treat tissue necrosis [40]. Additionally, olive oil contains several bioactive ingredients which enhance the regeneration of necrosed tissues [8,41–47]. Recently, a mixture of rosemary and chamomile oils with honey, induced efficient and rapid skin regeneration of equine-skin wounds experimentally and clinically [21]. In this study, we compared the healing efficacy of a natural composite containing rosemary oil, chamomile oil, sesame oil, olive oil and clover flower bee honey to other commercial products on thermally induced skin burns in rabbits.

2. Materials and Methods

2.1. Commercial Creames and Composite Preparation

Commercial creams used in this study were the MEBO®-cream (0.25% β-sitosterol, Julphar, Ras Al-Khaimah, United Arab Emirates) and DERMAZIN®-cream (1% silver sulfadiazine, SANDOZ, Cairo, Egypt). The composite (formulated in this study) consists of 80% (w/w) active ingredients and 20% (w/w) vaseline base. The active ingredients were a mixture of the following: sesame oil 30%, olive oil 10%, rosemary oil 10% and chamomile oil 10% (Alcaptin Pharm Co., Cairo, Egypt), and clover flower bee honey 20% (Agriculture Ministry, Giza, Egypt).

2.2. Composite Preparation

Firstly, honey was stirred on magnetic Stirrer (MGS-1C, Shaoxing, China) at 1500 rpm at 37 °C for 10 min. Then the oil mixtures were added drop by drop until complete mixing. Finally, vaseline (37 °C) was added slowly until complete mixing with the composite.

2.3. Experimental Design

Animal-handling procedures as well as sample collection and disposal were done according to the regulations of Institutional Animal Care and Use Committee (IACUC), with approval number: VUSC-004-1-22. It was planned to kill animals humanely if they showed "a generalized dermatitis" or accompanied by complications that cannot be treated. Ten healthy adult male New Zealand Rabbit were used. The mean body weight was 3.6 kg (range from 3.2 to 4 kg). Animals were housed in rabbit cages (one animal per cage) and fed with commercial rabbit diet (Super Rabbit, Egyptian European Company, Cairo, Egypt) while water was dispensed ad libitum along the period of the study. Animal acclimatization was continued for one week, then hair depletion was done using Veet™ (Veet, Cairo, Egypt) cream topically for three minutes. The experimental design is illustrated in Figure 1.

In the next day, anesthesia was induced in rabbits using xylazine and ketamine as method described by Oguntoye et al. [48]. Briefly, rabbits were premedicated first with xylazine (Xylaject®: 2% sol. Adwia Company, Cairo, Egypt) at a dose rate of 5 mg/kg. Anesthesia was induced with ketamine (Ketalar®: 5% sol. Amoun Company, Egypt) at a dose rate 35 mg/kg. All drugs were injected into *Longissimus dorsi* muscle at different locations. When the animal become anesthetized, four burn-wounds were created by aluminum stamp (80 °C/14 s) on the back of the animal by using electronic thermal aluminum stamp, manufactured locally as described by Knabl et al. [49] with some modifications by addition of electronic thermal controller (Figure 2).

Each wound from the created four wounds represents one of the following treatment groups; non-treated group, natural composite treated, MEBO® cream treated, and silver sulfadiazine® cream treated groups, respectively. The site of wounds was anatomically fixed in all rabbits and the distance between the two wounds in the same side was 11 cm, while the distance between wounds from right to left sides was 7 cm (Figure 3).

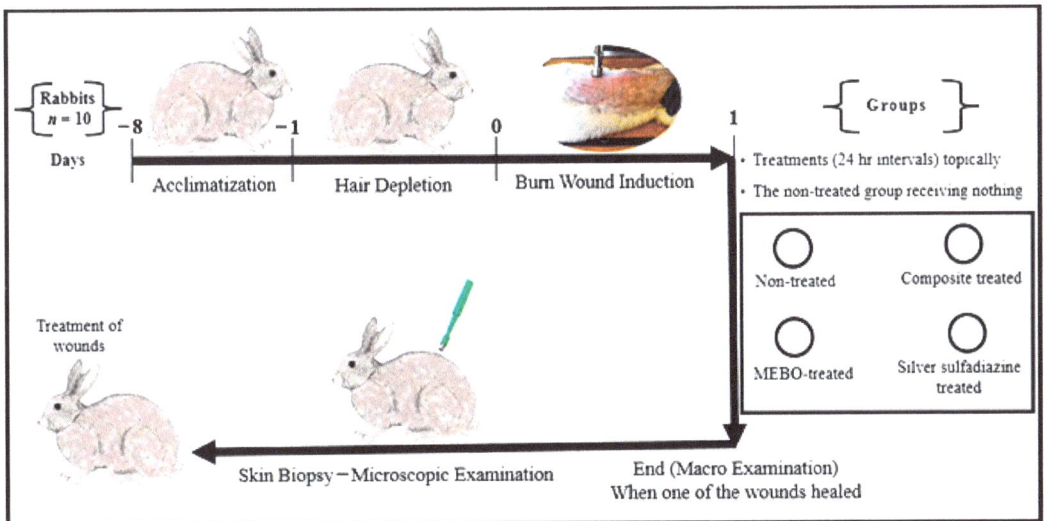

Figure 1. Infograph representing the experimental design. Acclimatization was continued for one week. Hair depletion was done using Veet™ cream topically for three minutes. Burn wound induction was done under the effect of general anaesthesia, four burn-wounds were created by aluminum stamp (80 °C/14 s) on the back of the animal using electronic thermal aluminum stamp represents one of the following treatment groups; non-treated group, natural composite treated group, MEBO® cream treated group, and silver sulfadiazine® cream treated group, respectively. Skin biopsies were collected from the central part of the wounds using disposable skin biopsy punches 10 mm under the effect of general anaesthesia.

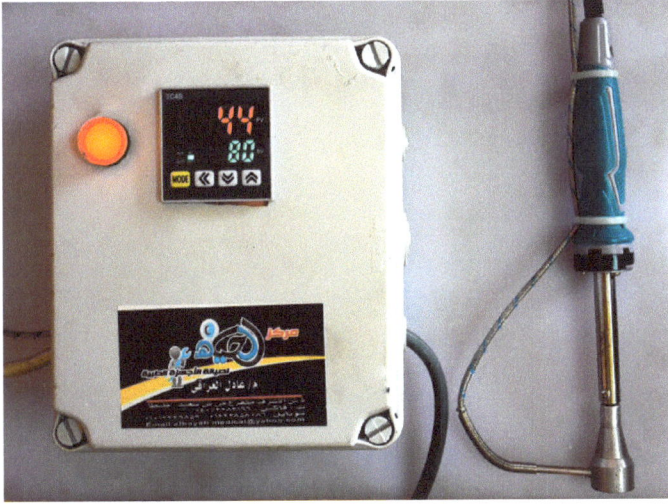

Figure 2. Adjustable electrical aluminum stamp for induction of thermal burn-wounds.

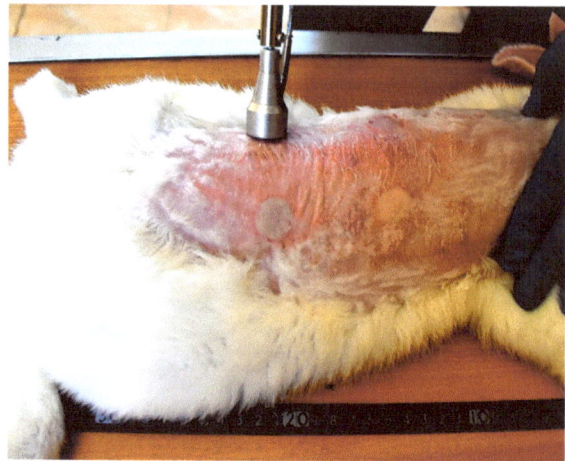

Figure 3. Induction of skin burns in adult New Zealand rabbit. Skin burns were induced using aluminum stamp; the contact area was 4 cm^2. The site of wounds was anatomically fixed in all rabbits and the distance between the two wounds in the same side was 11 cm, while the distance between wounds from right to left sides was 7 cm.

At the first day of burn induction, skin biopsies were taken from one rabbit at the center of the wound, by using disposable skin biopsy punches 10 mm (MentoK, Jaipur, India), under the effect of general anesthesia for histopathological evaluation of the wounds directly after burn induction. The other nine rabbits were used for the experiment. Treatments were applied once a day topically on the wound and the non-treated group received nothing. The experiment was terminated when one of the wounds appeared to be healed macroscopically. At the end of the experiment, skin biopsies were taken from the center of the wounds, by using disposable skin biopsy punches 10 mm (MentoK, India), under the effect of general anesthesia. After taking skin samples, all rabbits were subjected to intensive medical care to treat wounds created by the biopsy punches. Wounds were sutured and sprayed with betadine until complete healing and the animals were terminated by euthanization.

2.4. Histopathological Investigation

Samples were fixed with neutral buffered formalin 10% for 72 h then processed and sectioned at 3–5 um using Leica microtome. Tissues sections were stained with hematoxylin and eosin stain and the histological images were captured using Leica DMLB microscopes and Leica EC3 digital camera.

2.5. Morphometery

The morphometric evaluation was done according to methods described previously [50], with some modifications. Briefly, the images were taken with ×20 lens and saved in TIFF format. For each group, nine fields were taken (one field from each animal-skin sample). All fields were taken from the center of the wound. After the fields were saved, the Adobe photoshop program CS6 was used to improve them, using the lighting reference so that they all have the same quality. The full thickness of epidermis and the thickness of stratum corneum were calculated using ImageJ® (Bethesda, MD, USA) program and recorded in a Microsoft Excel spreadsheet.

2.6. Statistic Analysis

The data of epidermal measurements are presented as means ± standard error (S.E.) of the means. All morphometric data were subjected to One-way analysis of variance

(ANOVA) followed by Duncan's multiple range test for post hoc analysis using SPSS software, version 17 (IBM, Armonk, NY, USA). The significance level was set at $p \leq 0.05$.

3. Results

3.1. Pathological Evaluation of Skin Burns at the First Day of Induction

Grossly, circumscribed area of coagulative necrosis which was elevated above the skin surface and take a whitish color (Figure 3). Histopathologically, wounds were recorded as "second-degree burns" (superficial partial-thickness burns). Coagulative necrosis of both epidermal and dermal skin layers was found with a separation between epidermal and dermal layers, as well as denaturation of dermal collagens bundles (Figure 4A,B).

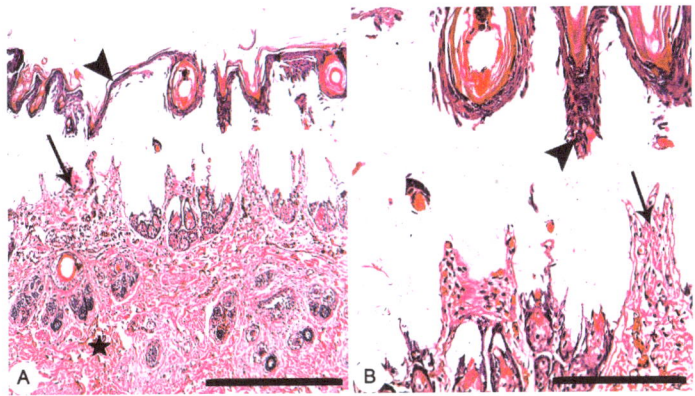

Figure 4. Skin, Rabbit. (**A**,**B**) Thermally induced skin burns using aluminum stamp (80 °C/ 14 s), showing second-degree burns which characterized by necrosis of both epidermal (arrowheads) and dermal (arrows) skin layers with a separation between epidermal and dermal layers, as well as denaturation of dermal collagens bundles (star). HE stain; Bars (**A**) 500 μm; (**B**) 100 μm.

3.2. Pathological Evaluation of Skin Burns at the End of the Experiment

Grossly, after 28 days of the treatment, a dry crust on the burn sites of the non-treated group were observed and a complete healing of the burn sites of the other groups were recorded (Figure 5).

Histopathologically, after 28 days of the treatment, non-treated group exhibited crusts on the surface of the skin. The skin was denuded from the epidermal layer in some parts with advancing epidermal tongue growing over the granulation tissues in other parts (Figure 6A). In composite cream treated group, a mature and complete epidermal skin-layers which covering the granulation tissue was recorded (Figure 6B). In MEBO® cream treated group, a complete epidermal skin-layers, but with a thin stratum corneum, covering the granulation tissue was found (Figure 6C). Finally, a complete epidermal layer, but with a thin stratum corneum, covering a granulation tissue was observed in silver sulfadiazine cream treated group (Figure 6D).

3.3. Morphometric Analysis

Table 1 and Figure 7 present the morphometric changes in the epidermal thickness of normal and different treated groups. According to the data shown, there was no significant differences in epidermal thickness between normal rabbit and composite- treated group. The epidermal thickness of composite-treated group was significantly higher than those of all other groups. Additionally, there was significant different between non-treated group, MEBO®-treated group and silver sulfadiazine-treated group (Figure 7A). Finally, the differences of the thickness of stratum corneum of both normal rabbit and composite-treated group was non-significant and both groups were highly significant than all other groups (Figure 7B).

Table 1. Epidermal thickness of normal rabbit skin and different treated groups (TG) in induced skin burns. Values are presented as mean ± SE ($n = 9$). Different letters (a, b, c, and d) in the same column indicate significant differences at $p < 0.05$.

Groups	Full Epidermal Thickness (μm)	Stratum Corneum Thickness (μm)
Normal skin	184.6 ± 5.09 [a]	22.8 ± 1.48 [a]
Non-treated	3.9 ± 2.63 [d]	0.5 ± 0.35 [c]
Composite-treated [1]	177.8 ± 3.39 [a]	20.8 ± 1.31 [a]
MEBO® cream-treated [2]	126.0 ± 2.59 [c]	5.0 ± 0.27 [b]
DERMAZIN®-treated [3]	139.0 ± 6.38 [b]	6.8 ± 0.21 [b]

[1] Composite cream: sesame oil 30%, olive oil 10%, rosemary oil 10% and chamomile oil 10% and clover flower bee honey 20%, and 20% (w/w) vaseline base. [2] MEBO®-cream = 0.25% β-sitosterol. [3] DERMAZIN®-cream = 1% silver sulfadiazine.

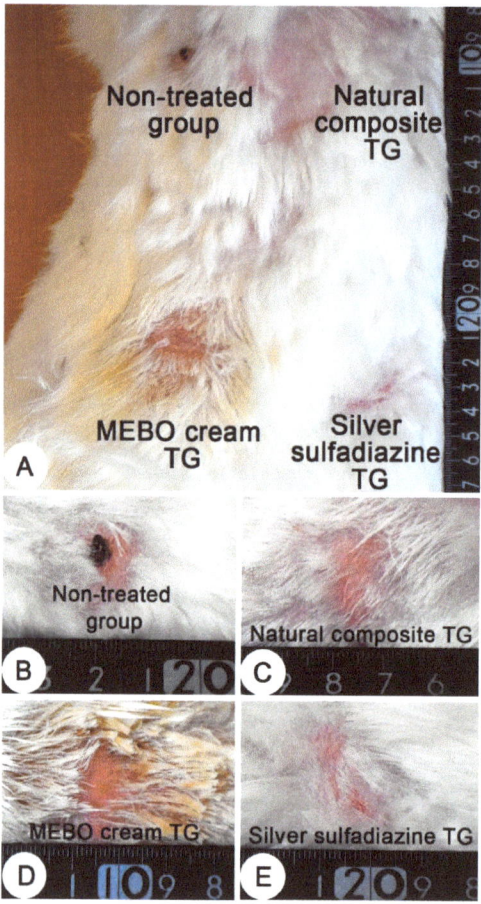

Figure 5. Skin, adult New Zealand rabbit. (**A**) Thermally induced skin burns after 28 days of treatment, showing the four burn sites in one animal. (**B–E**) a higher magnification of burn sites of figure A which representing the four treated groups. (**B**) dry crust on the burn site of the non-treated group. (**C–E**) complete healing of the burn sites of the treated groups. (**C**) composite cream treated group; (**D**) MEBO® cream treated group and (**E**) silver sulfadiazine cream treated group.

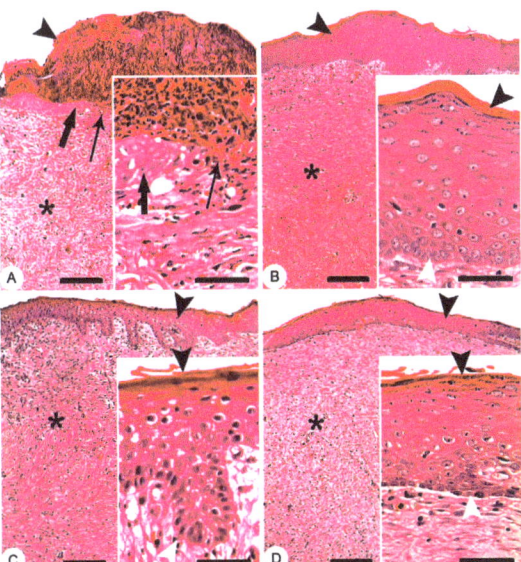

Figure 6. Skin, New Zealand rabbit. Histopathology of thermally induced skin burns after 28 days of treatment. (**A**) non-treated group showing crusts on the surface of the skin (arrowhead), denuded skin surface from the epidermal layer (thin arrow) and a granulation tissue (asterisk). Inset showing crawling of the epidermal cells (thick arrow) over the granulation tissues of the denuded skin (thin arrow). (**B**) composite cream treated group showing complete epidermal layer (arrowhead) covering a granulation tissue (asterisk). Inset showing mature and complete epidermal layers between the stratum corneum (black arrowhead) and stratum germinativum (white arrowhead). (**C**) MEBO® cream treated group showing complete epidermal layer (arrowhead) covering a granulation tissue (asterisk). Inset showing complete epidermal layers between a thin stratum corneum (black arrowhead) and stratum germinativum (white arrowhead). (**D**) silver sulfadiazine cream treated group showing complete epidermal layer (arrowhead) covering a granulation tissue (asterisk). Inset showing complete epidermal layers between a thin stratum corneum (black arrowhead) and stratum germinativum (white arrowhead). HE stain; Bars: main figures 200 µm, Inset 50 µm.

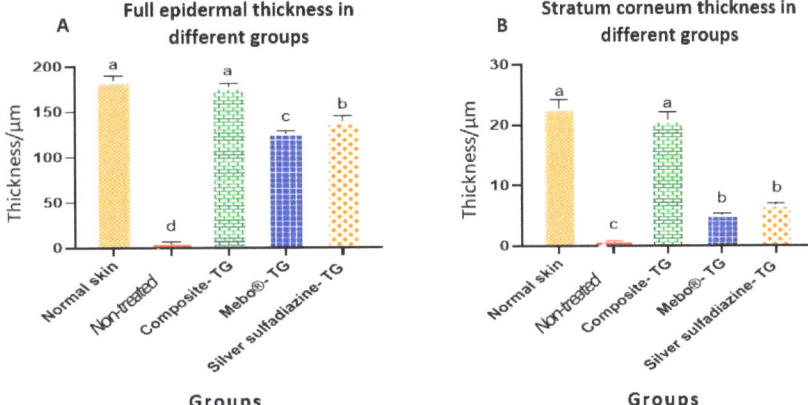

Figure 7. Full epidermal and stratum corneum thickness of normal rabbit skin and different treated groups of experimentally induced skin burns. The measured histological cuts per treatment = 9. Bars with different letters (a, b, c, and d) are significantly different at $p < 0.05$.

4. Discussion

Medication of skin burns are relatively too expensive, especially in poor countries; thus, a discovery of new compounds for skin protection and regeneration are still required [10]. Therefore, we tried to make our efforts to contribute in the discovery of new efficient and cheap phytogenic compounds to accelerate wound healing. This experiment was based on the fact that clover-flower bee honey, rosemary and chamomile oils accelerated wound healing in equines [21]. In this study, we have added sesame oil and olive oil to the above-mentioned composite to make a new composite that can be useful in the treatment of skin burns. Sesame oil is rich in many biological active ingredients especially β-sitosterol [7,8,37,51], which is the active ingredient of a commercially available cream (MEBO®-cream). Additionally, olive oil has been used in various previous studies investigating its role in the wound healing process [8,43,52,53].

Herein, the effect of our composite (sesame oil 30%, olive oil 10%, rosemary oil 10% and chamomile oil 10%, clover flower bee honey 20% and Vaseline base 20%) on the skin regeneration process was compared with the most famous commercially available creams used in the treatment of skin burns in Egypt, MEBO® and DERMAZIN®. MEBO® is composed mainly of 0.25% β-sitosterol in a base of sesame oil and beeswax [53], while DERMAZIN® is composed of 1% silver sulfadiazine, which was used previously in many studies on the matter of burn healing process [54–57].

Interestingly, thermally induced skin burns have been healed after 28 days of the treatment except the of negative control group (Figure 5). In all treated groups (except of the non-treated group), the healing process was grossly similar, but histologically, we can distinguish between the different treated groups according to the epidermal structures. In previous studies, MEBO® cream resulted in significant enhancement of wound healing in both healthy and immunocompromised dogs when compared to honey alone and the wound healing effect of MEBO® cream was superior to that of honey [7]. Additionally, silver sulfadiazine was subjected to many studies to evaluate its healing efficacy. It was revealed that silver sulfadiazine accelerated the healing process of burns [56,58]. On the other hand, some plant extracts like *Alpinia officinarum* (galangal) are significantly superior to silver sulfadiazine in the treatment of wound burns [55]. In this study, the healing efficacy of MEBO® cream, silver sulfadiazine cream and our composite were quite similar macroscopically (Figure 5). However, microscopically, the epidermal layer of composite cream treated groups was more mature than those of MEBO® cream and silver sulfadiazine treated groups (Figure 6). In addition, the morphometric analysis (Table 1 and Figure 7) showed that, epidermal thickness of the composite treated group was significantly higher than those of other treated groups. The thickness of stratum corneum of the composite treated wounds in addition to the arrangement and thickness of epidermal layers were quite similar to normal skin structures.

Although the bioactive substances of the natural composite were not analyzed (limitation of this study), the healing efficacy of the composite may be attributed to the nutrients and antibacterial potency of honey [59–61], growth promoters and nutrients of both rosemary and chamomile oils [62–64], anti-inflammatory and antioxidant properties of sesame oil [7] and vitamins and antioxidants in olive oil. The tested composite characterized by smooth and fast regeneration of the epidermal layers resulting in healthy and histologically uniformed epidermal layers which may be attributed to the several bioactive compounds which present in each component of the tested composite.

5. Conclusions

The non-treated group showed a slowed wound healing as compared to the other groups. However, the natural composite promotes the wound healing effectively, highlighting the potential use of natural compounds as effective and safe treatment of skin burns.

Author Contributions: Conceptualization, A.A., A.S. and S.E.H.; methodology, A.A., A.S. and S.E.H.; software, A.A.; validation, A.A., A.S., S.E.H. and A.A.S.; formal analysis, A.A.; resources, A.A.; data curation, A.A., A.S. and S.E.H.; writing—original draft preparation, A.A.; writing—review and editing, A.A., A.S., S.E.H. and A.A.S.; project administration, A.A.; funding acquisition, A.A. All authors have read and agreed to the published version of the manuscript.

Funding: This research was funded by University of Sadat City, Egypt, grant number 10.

Institutional Review Board Statement: The study was conducted in accordance with the regulations of Institutional Animal Care and Use Committee (IACUC), Faculty of Veterinary Medicine, University of Sadat city, with approval number: VUSC-004-1-22.

Informed Consent Statement: Not applicable.

Data Availability Statement: Not applicable.

Acknowledgments: We acknowledge all the former and present leaders of University of Sadat City and the former and present leaders of Faculty of Veterinary Medicine, University of Sadat City for facilitating all the University and College capabilities to complete this research. We also want to thank Nermeen B. El-Borai, Department of Forensic Medicine and Toxicology, Faculty of Veterinary Medicine, University of Sadat City, for here help in statistical analysis. Additionally, we would like to thank Asmaa Lotfy and veterinarian Naeima Othman, Department of pathology, Faculty of Veterinary Medicine, University of Sadat City for their technical assistant.

Conflicts of Interest: The authors declare no conflict of interest.

References

1. Forjuoh, S.N. Burns in low- and middle-income countries: A review of available literature on descriptive epidemiology, risk factors, treatment, and prevention. *Burns* **2006**, *32*, 529–537. [CrossRef] [PubMed]
2. Peck, M.D.; Kruger, G.E.; van der Merwe, A.E.; Godakumbura, W.; Ahuja, R.B. Burns and fires from non-electric domestic appliances in low and middle income countries: Part I. The scope of the problem. *Burns* **2008**, *34*, 303–311. [CrossRef]
3. World Health Organization. Burns. 2018. Available online: https://www.who.int/news-room/fact-sheets/detail/burns (accessed on 15 May 2022).
4. Mssillou, I.; Agour, A.; Slighoua, M.; Chebaibi, M.; Amrati, F.E.; Alshawwa, S.Z.; Kamaly, O.A.; El Moussaoui, A.; Lyoussi, B.; Derwich, E. Ointment-based vombination of *Dittrichia viscosa* L. and *Marrubium vulgare* L. accelerate burn wound healing. *Pharmaceuticals* **2022**, *15*, 289. [CrossRef] [PubMed]
5. Pavletic, M.M.; Trout, N.J. Bullet, bite, and burn wounds in dogs and cats. *Vet. Clin. Small Anim. Pract.* **2006**, *36*, 873–893. [CrossRef]
6. Schwartz, S.L.; Schick, A.E.; Lewis, T.P.; Loeffler, D. Dorsal thermal necrosis in dogs: Aretrospective analysis of 16 cases in the southwestern USA (2009–2016). *Vet. Dermatol.* **2018**, *29*, 139-e155. [CrossRef]
7. Alshehabat, M.; Hananeh, W.; Ismail, Z.B.; Rmilah, S.A.; Abeeleh, M.A. Wound healing in immunocompromised dogs: A comparison between the healing effects of moist exposed burn ointment and honey. *Vet. World* **2020**, *13*, 2793–2797. [CrossRef]
8. Przadka, P.; Kuberka, M.; Skrzypczak, P.; Kielbowicz, Z. Healing of a large skin defect in a dog with concurrent ozonated olive oil application. *J. Small Anim. Pract.* **2022**, *63*, 42. [CrossRef] [PubMed]
9. Jeschke, M.G.; van Baar, M.E.; Choudhry, M.A.; Chung, K.K.; Gibran, N.S.; Logsetty, S. Burn injury. *Nat. Rev. Dis. Primers* **2020**, *6*, 11. [CrossRef]
10. Heidari, M.; Bahramsoltani, R.; Abdolghaffari, A.H.; Rahimi, R.; Esfandyari, M.; Baeeri, M.; Hassanzadeh, G.; Abdollahi, M.; Farzaei, M.H. Efficacy of topical application of standardized extract of *Tragopogon graminifolius* in the healing process of experimental burn wounds. *J. Tradit. Complement. Med.* **2019**, *9*, 54–59. [CrossRef]
11. Van Yperen, D.T.; van Lieshout, E.M.M.; Nugteren, L.H.T.; Plaisier, A.C.; Verhofstad, M.H.J.; van der Vlies, C.H. Adherence to the emergency management of severe burns referral criteria in burn patients admitted to a hospital with or without a specialized burn center. *Burns* **2021**, *47*, 1810–1817. [CrossRef]
12. Arturson, G. Pathophysiology of the burn wound and pharmacological treatment. The Rudi Hermans Lecture, 1995. *Burns* **1996**, *22*, 255–274. [CrossRef]
13. Hargis, A.; Lewis, T. Full-thickness cutaneous burn in black-haired skin on the dorsum of the body of a Dalmation puppy. *Vet. Dermatol.* **1999**, *10*, 39–42. [CrossRef] [PubMed]
14. Sumner, J.P.; Pucheu-Haston, C.M.; Fowlkes, N.; Merchant, S. Dorsal skin necrosis secondary to a solar-induced thermal burn in a brown-coated dachshund. *Can. Vet. J.* **2016**, *57*, 305–308. [PubMed]
15. Magnusson, B.M.; Walters, K.A.; Roberts, M.S. Veterinary drug delivery: Potential for skin penetration enhancement. *Adv. Drug Deliv. Rev.* **2001**, *50*, 205–227. [CrossRef]
16. Thomas, G.W.; Rael, L.T.; Bar-Or, R.; Shimonkevitz, R.; Mains, C.W.; Slone, D.S.; Craun, M.L.; Bar-Or, D. Mechanisms of delayed wound healing by commonly used antiseptics. *J. Trauma Acute Care Surg.* **2009**, *66*, 82–91. [CrossRef]

17. Gupta, A.; Upadhyay, N.K.; Sawhney, R.; Kumar, R. A poly-herbal formulation accelerates normal and impaired diabetic wound healing. *Wound Repair Regen.* **2008**, *16*, 784–790. [CrossRef]
18. Bulut, S.P.; Gurbuzel, M.; Karabela, S.N.; Pence, H.H.; Aksaray, S.; Topal, U. The investigation of biochemical and microbiological properties of four different honey types produced in turkey and the comparison of their effects with silver sulfadiazine on wound healing in a rat model of burn injury. *Niger. J. Clin. Pract.* **2021**, *24*, 1694–1705. [CrossRef]
19. De Macedo, L.M.; Santos, E.M.D.; Militao, L.; Tundisi, L.L.; Ataide, J.A.; Souto, E.B.; Mazzola, P.G. Rosemary (*Rosmarinus officinalis* L., syn *Salvia rosmarinus* Spenn.) and its topical applications: A review. *Plants* **2020**, *9*, 651. [CrossRef]
20. Kazemian, H.; Ghafourian, S.; Sadeghifard, N.; Houshmandfar, R.; Badakhsh, B.; Taji, A.; Shavalipour, A.; Mohebi, R.; Ebrahim-Saraie, H.S.; Houri, H.; et al. In vivo antibacterial and wound healing activities of Roman Chamomile (*Chamaemelum nobile*). *Infect. Disord. Drug Targets* **2018**, *18*, 41–45. [CrossRef]
21. Anis, A.; Sharshar, A.; Hanbally, S.E.; Sadek, Y. A novel organic composite accelerates wound healing: Experimental and clinical study in equine. *J. Equine Vet. Sci.* **2021**, *99*, 103406. [CrossRef]
22. Vaghardoost, R.; Mousavi Majd, S.G.; Tebyanian, H.; Babavalian, H.; Malaei, L.; Niazi, M.; Javdani, A. The healing fffect of sesame oil, camphor and honey on second degree burn wounds in Rat. *World J. Plast. Surg.* **2018**, *7*, 67–71. [PubMed]
23. Auh, J.H.; Madhavan, J. Protective effect of a mixture of marigold and rosemary extracts on UV-induced photoaging in mice. *Biomed. Pharm.* **2021**, *135*, 111178. [CrossRef] [PubMed]
24. Nakagawa, S.; Hillebrand, G.G.; Nunez, G. *Rosmarinus officinalis* L. (Rosemary) extracts containing carnosic acid and carnosol are potent quorum sensing inhibitors of *Staphylococcus aureus* virulence. *Antibiotics* **2020**, *9*, 149. [CrossRef] [PubMed]
25. Sanchez-Marzo, N.; Perez-Sanchez, A.; Barrajon-Catalan, E.; Castillo, J.; Herranz-Lopez, M.; Micol, V. Rosemary diterpenes and flavanone aglycones provide improved genoprotection against UV-dnduced DNA damage in a human skin cell model. *Antioxidants* **2020**, *9*, 255. [CrossRef] [PubMed]
26. Pazyar, N.; Yaghoobi, R.; Rafiee, E.; Mehrabian, A.; Feily, A. Skin wound healing and phytomedicine: A review. *Ski. Pharmacol. Physiol.* **2014**, *27*, 303–310. [CrossRef] [PubMed]
27. Ariffin, N.H.M.; Hasham, R. Potential dermatological application on Asian plants. *Biotechnol. Bioprocess Eng.* **2016**, *21*, 337–354. [CrossRef]
28. Ojeda-Sana, A.M.; van Baren, C.M.; Elechosa, M.A.; Juárez, M.A.; Moreno, S. New insights into antibacterial and antioxidant activities of rosemary essential oils and their main components. *Food Control* **2013**, *31*, 189–195. [CrossRef]
29. Fernández-Ochoa, Á.; Borras-Linares, I.; Pérez-Sánchez, A.; Barrajón-Catalán, E.; Gonzalez-Alvarez, I.; Arráez-Román, D.; Micol, V.; Segura-Carretero, A. Phenolic compounds in rosemary as potential source of bioactive compounds against colorectal cancer: In situ absorption and metabolism study. *J. Funct. Foods* **2017**, *33*, 202–210. [CrossRef]
30. O'G'Li, F.J.S. Chamomile: A herbal medicine of the past with bright future. *Eur. Int. J. Multidiscip. Res. Manag. Stud.* **2022**, *2*, 251–254.
31. Marderosian, A.D.; Liberti, L.E.; Krikorian, A.D. Natural product medicine: A scientific guide to foods, drugs, cosmetics. *Q. Rev. Biol.* **1989**, *64*, 106–107. Available online: https://www.journals.uchicago.edu/doi/abs/10.1086/416216 (accessed on 31 May 2022).
32. Thornfeldt, C. Cosmeceuticals containing herbs: Fact, fiction, and future. *Dermatol. Surg.* **2005**, *31*, 873–881. [CrossRef] [PubMed]
33. Garbuio, D.C.; Ribeiro, V.D.S.; Hamamura, A.C.; Faustino, A.; Freitas, L.A.P.; Viani, G.; Carvalho, E.C. A Chitosan-coated chamomile microparticles formulation to prevent radiodermatitis in breast: A double-blinded, controlled, randomized, Phase II clinical trial. *Am. J. Clin. Oncol.* **2022**, *45*, 183–189. [CrossRef] [PubMed]
34. Ferreira, E.B.; Ciol, M.A.; de Meneses, A.G.; Bontempo, P.S.M.; Hoffman, J.M.; Reis, P. Chamomile gel versus urea cream to prevent acute radiation dermatitis in head and neck cancer patients: Results from a preliminary clinical trial. *Integr. Cancer* **2020**, *19*, 1534735420962174. [CrossRef] [PubMed]
35. Ogawa, T.; Ishitsuka, Y.; Nakamura, Y.; Okiyama, N.; Watanabe, R.; Fujisawa, Y.; Fujimoto, M. Honey and chamomile activate keratinocyte antioxidative responses via the KEAP1/NRF2 system. *Clin. Cosmet. Investig. Derm.* **2020**, *13*, 657–660. [CrossRef]
36. El-Salamouni, N.S.; Ali, M.M.; Abdelhady, S.A.; Kandil, L.S.; Elbatouti, G.A.; Farid, R.M. Evaluation of chamomile oil and nanoemulgels as a promising treatment option for atopic dermatitis induced in rats. *Expert Opin. Drug Deliv.* **2020**, *17*, 111–122. [CrossRef]
37. Ebrahimpour, N.; Mehrabani, M.; Iranpour, M.; Kordestani, Z.; Mehrabani, M.; Nematollahi, M.H.; Asadipour, A.; Raeiszadeh, M.; Mehrbani, M. The efficacy of a traditional medicine preparation on second-degree burn wounds in rats. *J. Ethnopharmacol.* **2020**, *252*, 112570. [CrossRef]
38. Saporito, F.; Sandri, G.; Bonferoni, M.C.; Rossi, S.; Boselli, C.; Icaro Cornaglia, A.; Mannucci, B.; Grisoli, P.; Vigani, B.; Ferrari, F. Essential oil-loaded lipid nanoparticles for wound healing. *Int. J. Nanomed.* **2018**, *13*, 175–186. [CrossRef]
39. Bayir, Y.; Un, H.; Ugan, R.A.; Akpinar, E.; Cadirci, E.; Calik, I.; Halici, Z. The effects of beeswax, olive oil and butter impregnated bandage on burn wound healing. *Burns* **2019**, *45*, 1410–1417. [CrossRef]
40. Gupta, E. β-Sitosterol: Predominant phytosterol of therapeutic potential. In *Innovations in Food Technology*; Springer: Singapore, 2020; pp. 465–477.
41. Solt Kirca, A.; Kanza Gul, D. Effects of olive oil on *Striae Gravidarum* in primiparous women: A randomized controlled clinical study. *Altern. Health Med.* **2022**, *28*, 34–39.

42. Shalaby, K. Effect of olive oil acidity on skin delivery of diclofenac: In vitro evaluation and ex vivo skin permeability studies. *J. Biomed. Nanotechnol.* **2022**, *18*, 234–242. [CrossRef]
43. Massoud, D.; Fouda, M.M.A.; Sarhan, M.; Salama, S.G.; Khalifa, H.S. Topical application of aloe gel and/or olive oil combination promotes the wound healing properties of streptozotocin-induced diabetic rats. *Environ. Sci. Pollut. Res. Int.* **2022**, *29*, 59727–59735. [CrossRef] [PubMed]
44. Gul, U.; Khan, M.I.; Madni, A.; Sohail, M.F.; Rehman, M.; Rasul, A.; Peltonen, L. Olive oil and clove oil-based nanoemulsion for topical delivery of terbinafine hydrochloride: In vitro and ex vivo evaluation. *Drug Deliv.* **2022**, *29*, 600–612. [CrossRef] [PubMed]
45. Donato-Trancoso, A.; Correa Atella, G.; Romana-Souza, B. Dietary olive oil intake aggravates psoriatic skin inflammation in mice via Nrf2 activation and polyunsaturated fatty acid imbalance. *Int. Immunopharmacol.* **2022**, *108*, 108851. [CrossRef] [PubMed]
46. Baptista, S.; Pereira, J.R.; Gil, C.V.; Torres, C.A.V.; Reis, M.A.M.; Freitas, F. Development of olive oil and alpha-tocopherol containing emulsions stabilized by FucoPol: Rheological and textural analyses. *Polymers* **2022**, *14*, 2349. [CrossRef]
47. Alnemer, F.; Aljohani, R.; Alajlan, A.; Aljohani, M.; Alozaib, I.; Masuadi, E.; Omair, A.; Al Jasser, M.I. The use of olive oil for skin health in a Saudi population: A cross-sectional study. *Derm. Rep.* **2022**, *14*, 9364. [CrossRef]
48. Oguntoye, C.; Oke, B. A comparison of xylazine/ketamine, diazepam/ketamine and acepromazine/ketamine anaesthesia in rabbit. *Sokoto J. Vet. Sci.* **2014**, *12*, 21–25. [CrossRef]
49. Knabl, J.S.; Bayer, G.S.; Bauer, W.A.; Schwendenwein, I.; Dado, P.F.; Kucher, C.; Horvat, R.; Turkof, E.; Schossmann, B.; Meissl, G. Controlled partial skin thickness burns: An animal model for studies of burnwound progression. *Burns* **1999**, *25*, 229–235. [CrossRef]
50. Monaretti, G.L.; Costa, M.C.F.; Rocha, L.B.; Cintra, M.M.M.; da Cunha, M.T.R.; Pinheiro, N.M.; Noites, A.; Mendonca, A.C. Effect of capacitive radiofrequency on the dermis of the abdominal region. *Lasers Med. Sci.* **2022**, *37*, 619–625. [CrossRef]
51. Hammam, W.E.; Gad, A.M.; Gad, M.K.; Kirollos, F.N.; Yassin, N.A.; Tantawi, M.E.E.; El Hawary, S.S.E. *Pyrus communis* L. (Pear) and *Malus domestica* Borkh. (apple) leaves lipoidal extracts as sources for beta-sitosterol rich formulae and their wound healing evaluation. *Nat. Prod. Res. online ahead of print.* **2022**. [CrossRef]
52. Moni, S.S.; Tripathi, P.; Sultan, M.H.; Alshahrani, S.; Alqahtani, S.S.; Madkhali, O.A.; Bakkari, M.A.; Pancholi, S.S.; Elmobark, M.E.; Jabeen, A.; et al. Wound-healing and cytokine-modulating potential of medicinal oil formulation comprising leaf extract of *Murraya koenigii* and olive oil. *Braz. J. Biol.* **2022**, *82*, e256158. [CrossRef]
53. Taheri, M.; Amiri-Farahani, L.; Haghani, S.; Shokrpour, M.; Shojaii, A. The effect of olive cream on pain and healing of caesarean section wounds: A randomised controlled clinical trial. *J. Wound Care* **2022**, *31*, 244–253. [CrossRef] [PubMed]
54. Devi, M.V.; Poornima, V.; Sivagnanam, U.T. Wound healing in second-degree burns in rats treated with silver sulfadiazine: A systematic review and meta-analysis. *J. Wound Care* **2022**, *31*, S31–S45. [CrossRef] [PubMed]
55. Kadam, K.; Kiyan, S.; Uyanikgil, Y.; Karabey, F.; Cetin, E.O. Investigation of acute effects of topical *Alpinia officinarum* (galangal) treatment in experimental contact type burns and comparison with topical silver sulfadiazine treatment. *Ulus Travma Acil Cerrahi Derg.* **2022**, *28*, 15–26. [CrossRef] [PubMed]
56. Singh, R.; Roopmani, P.; Chauhan, M.; Basu, S.M.; Deeksha, W.; Kazem, M.D.; Hazra, S.; Rajakumara, E.; Giri, J. Silver sulfadiazine loaded core-shell airbrushed nanofibers for burn wound healing application. *Int. J. Pharm.* **2022**, *613*, 121358. [CrossRef] [PubMed]
57. Wang, J.; Yang, B.; Zhang, X.H.; Liu, S.H.; Wu, W. The effectiveness of silver-containing hydrofiber dressing compared with topical silver sulfadiazine cream in pediatric patients with deep partial-thickness burns: A retrospective review. *Wound Manag. Prev.* **2022**, *68*, 29–36. [CrossRef]
58. Al-Arjan, W.S.; Khan, M.U.A.; Almutairi, H.H.; Alharbi, S.M.; Razak, S.I.A. pH-Responsive PVA/BC-f-GO Dressing materials for burn and chronic wound healing with curcumin release kinetics. *Polymers* **2022**, *14*, 949. [CrossRef]
59. Albaridi, N.A. Antibacterial potency of honey. *Int. J. Microbiol.* **2019**, *2019*, 2464507. [CrossRef]
60. Algethami, J.S.; El-Wahed, A.A.A.; Elashal, M.H.; Ahmed, H.R.; Elshafiey, E.H.; Omar, E.M.; Naggar, Y.A.; Algethami, A.F.; Shou, Q.; Alsharif, S.M.; et al. Bee pollen: Clinical trials and patent applications. *Nutrients* **2022**, *14*, 2858. [CrossRef]
61. El-Seedi, H.R.; El-Wahed, A.A.A.; Zhao, C.; Saeed, A.; Zou, X.; Guo, Z.; Hegazi, A.G.; Shehata, A.A.; El-Seedi, H.H.R.; Algethami, A.F.; et al. A Spotlight on the Egyptian honeybee (*Apis mellifera lamarckii*). *Animals* **2022**, *12*, 2749. [CrossRef]
62. Ghazalah, A.; Ali, A. Rosemary leaves as a dietary supplement for growth in broiler chickens. *Int. J. Poult. Sci.* **2008**, *7*, 234–239. [CrossRef]
63. Das, S.; Horváth, B.; Šafranko, S.; Jokić, S.; Széchenyi, A.; Kőszegi, T. Antimicrobial activity of chamomile essential oil: Effect of different formulations. *Molecules* **2019**, *24*, 4321. [CrossRef] [PubMed]
64. Shehata, A.A.; Yalçın, S.; Latorre, J.D.; Basiouni, S.; Attia, Y.A.; Abd El-Wahab, A.; Visscher, C.; El-Seedi, H.R.; Huber, C.; Hafez, H.M.; et al. Probiotics, prebiotics, and phytogenic substances for optimizing gut health in poultry. *Microorganisms* **2022**, *10*, 395. [CrossRef] [PubMed]

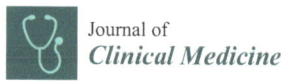

Article

The Impact of Antiseptic-Loaded Bacterial Nanocellulose on Different Biofilms—An Effective Treatment for Chronic Wounds?

Hanna Luze [1,*,†], Ives Bernardelli de Mattos [2,†,‡], Sebastian Philipp Nischwitz [1], Martin Funk [3], Alexandru Cristian Tuca [1] and Lars-Peter Kamolz [1,4,5]

1. Division of Plastic, Aesthetic and Reconstructive Surgery, Department of Surgery, Medical University of Graz, Auenbruggerplatz 29/2, 8036 Graz, Austria
2. Fraunhofer Institute for Silicate Research ISC, Translational Center Regenerative Therapies, 97070 Würzburg, Germany
3. EVOMEDIS GmbH, 8036 Graz, Austria
4. COREMED—Cooperative Centre for Regenerative Medicine, Joanneum Research Forschungsgesellschaft mbH, 8010 Graz, Austria
5. Research Unit for Safety in Health c/o Division of Plastic, Aesthetic and Reconstructive Surgery, Department of Surgery, Medical University of Graz, 8036 Graz, Austria
* Correspondence: hanna.luze@medunigraz.at; Tel.: +43-316-385-30445
† These authors contributed equally to this work.
‡ Ives Bernardelli de Mattos is co-first author.

Abstract: Introduction: Pathogenic biofilms are an important factor for impaired wound healing, subsequently leading to chronic wounds. Nonsurgical treatment of chronic wound infections is limited to the use of conventional systemic antibiotics and antiseptics. Wound dressings based on bacterial nanocellulose (BNC) are considered a promising approach as an effective carrier for antiseptics. The aim of the present study was to investigate the antimicrobial activity of antiseptic-loaded BNC against in vitro biofilms. **Materials and Methods**: BNC was loaded with the commercially available antiseptics Prontosan® and Octenisept®. The silver-based dressing Aquacel®Ag Extra was used as a positive control. The biofilm efficacy of the loaded BNC sheets was tested against an in vitro 24-hour biofilm of *Staphylococcus aureus* and *Candida albicans* and a 48-hour biofilm of *Pseudomonas aeruginosa*. In vivo tests using a porcine excisional wound model was used to analyze the effect of a prolonged treatment with the antiseptics on the healing process. **Results**: We observed complete eradication of *S. aureus* biofilm in BNC loaded with Octenisept® and *C. albicans* biofilm for BNC loaded with Octenisept® or Prontosan®. Treatment with unloaded BNC also resulted in a statistically significant reduction in bacterial cell density of *S. aureus* compared to untreated biofilm. No difference on the wound healing outcome was observed for the wounds treated for seven days using BNC alone in comparison to BNC combined with Prontosan® or with Octenisept®. **Conclusions**: Based on these results, antiseptic-loaded BNC represents a promising and effective approach for the treatment of biofilms. Additionally, the prolonged exposure to the antiseptics does not affect the healing outcome. Prevention and treatment of chronic wound infections may be feasible with this novel approach and may even be superior to existing modalities.

Keywords: antimicrobial dressings; antiseptic; bacterial nanocellulose; biofilm; chronic wounds

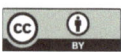

1. Introduction

The biological process of successful wound healing is achieved through four precisely programmed, consecutive phases: hemostasis, inflammation, proliferation, and remodeling [1]. Chronic wounds are wounds that fail to progress through the normal consecutive phases of wound healing in an orderly and timely manner. They represent a major burden to patients, healthcare providers and healthcare systems [2]. While wounds may be colonized with a variety of microorganisms, tissue invasion or damage does not happen necessarily [3]. Characterization of this biofilm includes a variety of techniques ranging from older established methods (e.g., wound swabs, counting of bacterial colonies) to modern technologies such as fluorescent labeling and mathematical predictive modeling [4].

Shifts in the colonization flora, however, may cause pathogenic biofilms, which may be considered one of the most important factors contributing to pathological wound healing in addition to numerous potential factors like the patient's age, nutritional status, or presence of a chronic disease or immunocompromised state [1,2]. The presence of pathogenic biofilm may also be accompanied with infection, causing local symptoms such as swelling, erythema, pain or heat [3,5].

Pathogenic biofilms usually consist of 10–20% pathogenic microbes, bacteria or fungi, that infect or invade the wound bed and 80–90% self-produced, extracellular polymeric substance [6]. Several genetic and biochemical effects within a pathogenic biofilm result in more vigorous immune responses, consequently leading to chronic inflammation compared to nonpathogenic biofilms that are effectively controlled and ultimately removed by the body's own clearing mechanisms [7]. Pathogenic biofilms are homogeneously distributed throughout the wound bed, impeding their identification and initiation of targeted therapeutic intervention [2].

While surgical debridement is an effective option in the reduction and eradication of bacterial load [8], nonsurgical attempts to eradicate pathogenic biofilms and treat chronic wound infections are limited to the use of conventional antibiotics and antiseptics to date [6].

The use of bacterial nanocellulose (BNC) as carriers for various "active" substances might be a clinically feasible approach to address this problem. This biomaterial meets several desirable characteristics of an "ideal" wound dressing such as being non-adhesive, reducing the number of dressing changes, allowing pH modulation of the wound bed [9] or providing a moisture balance and cooling effect [10]. In this context, BNC-based wound dressings are considered a suitable carrier for different commercially available antiseptics to directly inhibit bacterial growth [11,12]. The continuous and therapeutic release of active ingredients observed in BNC-based dressings is considered beneficial for wound treatment applications due to the homeostasis of steady concentrations over the entire treatment period [11]. The present study aimed to investigate the antimicrobial activity of antiseptic-loaded BNC against in vitro biofilms of Gram-positive and -negative bacteria as well as fungi. Furthermore, an in vivo test was proposed aiming to assess the effect of a prolonged exposure of antiseptics on the wound healing outcome.

2. Materials and Methods

Epicite^{hydro}® 10 × 10 cm sheets (QRSkin GmbH, Würzburg, Germany; Ref-No. 800003-M02B) were used as the BNC matrix carrier for application in the in vitro biofilm models. BNC was loaded with the commercially available polyhexanide (PHMB)-based antiseptic Prontosan® (B. Braun Melsungen Ag, Melsungen, Germany) or the octenidine-based antiseptic Octenisept® (Schülke & Mayr GmbH, Norderstedt, Germany) as described by Bernardelli et al. [11,12]. The silver-containing dressing Aquacel®Ag Extra (ConvaTech Group, United Kingdom) was used as a positive control, since this dressing is known for good results against microorganisms capable of producing biofilms [13]. The effect of loaded BNC on the biofilm was tested against a 24-hour biofilm of Gram-positive bacteria (*Staphylococcus aureus*) as well as fungi (*Candida albicans*) and a 48-hour biofilm of Gram-negative bacteria (*Pseudomonas aeruginosa*). A biofilm assay that was left untreated was used as a negative control.

2.1. 24-Hour CDC Bioreactor Model—S. aureus

The biofilm model that was used for these experiments was created according to the adapted ASTM International Standard (E2647-13). In short, an overnight culture of *S. aureus* (ATCC 6538) was set up by inoculation of 10 mL of Tryptone Soya Broth (TSB) with a single colony of the strain. The inoculated strain was incubated at 37 °C and 125 rpm in an orbital shaking incubator. The overnight culture of *S. aureus* was then adjusted to 0.5 McFarland

(~1 × 10⁸ colony-forming unit (CFU)/mL) in TSB. Then, 1 mL of the adjusted culture was used to inoculate the CDC bioreactor, which was made up to a final volume of 300 mL of TSB. The CDC bioreactor was incubated in batch phase at 37 °C and 65 rpm for 24 h. After 24 h, each epicite^hydro® dressing was placed in 100 mL of Prontosan® and Octenisept® for 30 min at room temperature. The process of loading the BNC was previously described by our group in 2019 [12]. Coupons were then briefly washed in Phosphate-Buffered Saline (PBS), then added in triplicate and incubated at 37 °C for 24 h. After 24 h of exposure, coupons were removed from the wells, added to 10 mL of Dey Engley neutralizing broth (Sigma-Aldrich, MA, USA) and sonicated for 30 min at full power. Each tube was briefly vortexed prior to sampling. Samples were added to 96-well plates, serial diluted in a ratio of 1:10 in PBS and plated onto Tryptone Soya Agar (TSA) in duplicate by pipetting 50 µL onto each half and spreading. Well plates were incubated overnight at 37 °C before enumeration of colony counts.

2.2. Drip-Flow Bioreactor—P. aeruginosa

Preparation of the drip-flow bioreactor was performed by adding a clean borosilicate microscope slide to each channel of the bioreactor prior to autoclavation at 121 °C for 15 min. An overnight inoculum was set up by inoculation of 10 mL of TSB with a single colony of *P. aeruginosa* (ATCC 700888) and incubation at 37 °C and 125 rpm. The overnight culture was adjusted to 0.5 McFarland (~1 × 10⁸ CFU/mL) on the following day. Each channel of the drip-flow bioreactor was clamped to stop flow, prior to adding 15 mL 3 g/L of TSB and 1 mL of adjusted culture to each channel. The drip-flow bioreactor was incubated for 6 h in batch phase and connected to a nutrient flow of 270 mg/L TSB at 50 mL/hour per channel in the following.

Epicite^hydro® dressing was placed in 100 mL of Prontosan® and Octenisept® for 30 min at room temperature. Loaded epicite^hydro® dressings were then added to each of the biofilm coated microscope slides in triplicate. The drip-flow bioreactor was reconnected to the carboy and operated for another 24 h. After the challenge period, each microscope slide was scraped into 45 mL of the appropriate neutralizer in a sterile 100 mL beaker. The slide was washed with 5 mL of neutralizer to ensure the removal of the whole biofilm. Each sample was homogenized for 30 s, serial diluted 1:10 in PBS and plated in duplicate onto TSA by pipetting 50 µL onto each side of a 2-compartment plate. Well plates were incubated overnight at 37 °C before enumeration of colony counts.

2.3. 24-Hour CDC Bioreactor Model—C. albicans

Two overnight cultures of *C. albicans* (ATCC 10231) were set up by inoculation of 10 mL of Sabouraud Dextrose Broth (SDB) with a single colony of the strain. The inoculated strain was incubated at 37 °C and 125 rpm in an orbital shaking incubator. The overnight cultures of *C. albicans* were then centrifuged at 5600 rpm, whereby the supernatants were discarded and resuspended in 1 mL of fresh SDB to inoculate the CDC bioreactor in the following. The CDC bioreactor was made up to a final volume of 300 mL of SDB and incubated in batch phase at 30 °C and 125 rpm for 24 h. After 24 h, the rods were washed twice in PBS and individual coupons were placed into 12-well plates. Each epicite^hydro® dressing was placed in 100 mL of Prontosan® and Octenisept® for 30 min at room temperature. A 2.5 cm × 5.0 cm section of the loaded dressings was added to each coupon in triplicate, and incubated for 24 h at 30 °C. After 24 h of exposure, coupons were removed from the wells and added to 10 mL of Dey Engley neutralizing broth and sonicated at full power for 30 min. Each tube was briefly vortexed prior to sample taking. Samples were added to 96-well plates, serial diluted 1:10 in PBS and plated onto SDB in duplicate by pipetting 50 µL onto each half and spreading. Well plates were incubated for 48 h at 30 °C before enumeration of colony counts.

2.4. Neutralizer Effectiveness Validation Assay

A neutralizer effectiveness validation assay was conducted using a broad-spectrum neutralizer (+saponin for Prontosan® WIF: EN 1276—2009) and Dey Engley neutralizing broth. An overnight culture of *P. aeruginosa* (ATCC 700888) was set up as described in Section 2.2.

The following day, Octenisept® was mixed at a ratio of 1:1 with the broad-spectrum neutralizer and Dey Engley neutralizing broth while Prontosan® was mixed at a ratio of 1:1 with the broad-spectrum neutralizer and saponin. A neutralizer toxicity control and a growth control of TSB only were included as well. After incubation for 10 min, the overnight culture of *P. aeruginosa* was adjusted to 0.5 McFarland (~1×10^8 CFU/mL) and added to the solutions at a final concentration of 1×10^6 CFU/mL prior to another incubation for 30 min. Solutions were then briefly vortexed, serial diluted 1:10 in PBS and plated out in duplicate, by pipetting 50 µL onto each half of a TSA plate and spreading. TSA well plates were incubated overnight at 37 °C before enumeration of colony counts.

2.5. In Vivo Tests

To assess if the healing process is affected by a prolonged treatment using octenidine-based and PHMB-based antiseptics, a porcine excisional wound model was used. The in vivo procedure was approved by The Animal Care and Use Committee (Veterinary University Vienna, Austrian Ministry of Science and Research). All the animals were treated in accordance with the recommendations of GV SOLAS (Gesellschaft für Versuchstierkunde/Society of Laboratory Animal Science, Germany). Using an electric dermatome, and under anesthesia and analgesia, 3×3-cm-sized wounds were generated in the dorsal part of two 3 month-old female domestic pigs (*Sus domesticus*; hybrid from Deutsche Landrasse and Deutsches Edelschwein) weighing 34 kg at the start of the experiments. The dermatome was set to excise 1.2 mm depth wounds, in order to mimic deep-partial burn wounds. To treat the wounds, 10×10 cm epicite^hydro® dressings were placed in kidney basins containing 5 times the BNC water content volume (100 mL per dressing) of Octenisept® and Prontosan® [11,12]. The dressings were then incubated for 30 min and 5×5 cm pieces were placed over the wound bed, to cover the wound completely. A total of 32 wounds, divided in the two animals, were treated using this approach. Twelve wounds were treated using epicite^hydro incubated with Octenisept®, and 12 were treated with the combination with Prontosan®. As a control, 8 wounds, 4 in each animal, were treated solely using the epicite^hydro dressings. The animals were treated for 7 days and euthanized under deep anesthesia. Then, 5×5 cm of the tissue comprising the wounds were extracted. The tissues were excised above the superficial fascia layer and placed in formaldehyde. During the entire procedure, photo documentation for macroscopical analysis was performed. The samples were sent to TPL path Labs GmbH (Germany), where slides were mounted, and samples were stained with Hematoxylin and Eosin (H&E). From each wound, two slides were prepared and analyzed blindly by a histopathologist. Several morphometric wound healing parameters were analyzed using the software Zen 3.3 blue edition (Zeiss Microscopy, Jena, Germany), including area, average thickness, and percentage of re-epithelialization for the regenerated epidermis and average thickness for the regenerated dermis.

2.6. Statistical Analysis

Raw data counts were put into Microsoft Excel and the CFU/mL was calculated. One-way ANOVA was performed as the means of inferential statistics using GraphPad Prism 7 software (GraphPad Software, Inc., San Diego, CA, USA). All statistical tests were two-tailed, and differences were considered statistically significant when $p < 0.05$.

3. Results

3.1. 24-Hour CDC Bioreactor Model—S. aureus

After a 24-h treatment of the *S. aureus* biofilms with unloaded epicite[hydro®] dressings, a bacterial density of 2.03×10^5 CFU/mL was observed. In comparison, the untreated biofilm showed a bacterial density of 1.31×10^7 CFU/mL. Treatment with unloaded epicite[hydro®] dressings therefore resulted in a statistically significant 2.0 log reduction in bacterial density ($p = 0.0055$). Biofilms treated with epicite[hydro®] loaded with Prontosan® showed a bacterial density 5.17×10^3 CFU/mL, exhibiting a statistically significant 4.9 log reduction in bacterial density ($p = 0.0055$). In biofilms treated with epicite[hydro®] loaded with Octenisept® or the positive control Aquacel® Ag Extra, no colonies were observed, exhibiting a 7.3 log reduction in bacterial cell density ($p = 0.0001$). The bacterial density reduction of *S. aureus* with all test dressings is displayed in Figure 1.

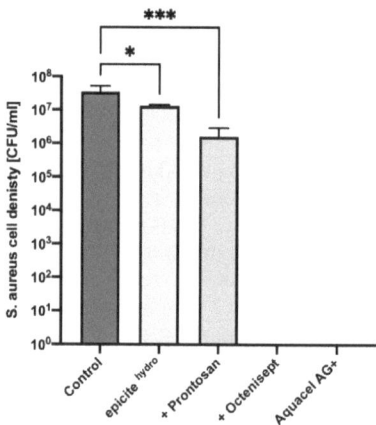

Figure 1. Log_{10} cell density of *S. aureus* (ATCC 6538) 24-h biofilm following 24-h treatment with the test dressings. All dressings were tested in triplicate. Error bars represent standard deviation of the mean. Asterisks represent the significant difference between the samples and the untreated control ($p = 0.0055$).

3.2. Drip-Flow Bioreactor—P. aeruginosa

After a 24-hour treatment of the *P. aeruginosa* biofilms with unloaded epicite[hydro®] dressings, a bacterial density of 1.43×10^9 CFU/mL was observed. In comparison, the untreated biofilm showed a similar bacterial density of 7.47×10^8 CFU/mL. Compared to the untreated biofilm, a 0.3 log increase in biofilm density was observed after the treatment with unloaded epicite[hydro®] dressings ($p = 0.033$). Biofilms treated with epicite[hydro®] loaded with Prontosan® or Octenisept® showed a bacterial cell density of 1.63×10^6 CFU/mL and 1.88×10^6 CFU/mL, respectively. In comparison to treatment with unloaded epicite[hydro®] exclusively, 2.7 log ($p = 0.0006$) and 2.6 log ($p = 0.0006$) reductions in biofilm density were observed, respectively. Treatment with the positive control Aquacel® Ag Extra showed a bacterial density of 3.34×10^6 CFU/mL ($p = 0.0019$), exhibiting a 2.3 log reduction when compared to epicite[hydro®] ($p = 0.003$). The bacterial density reduction of *P. aeruginosa* with all test dressings is displayed in Figure 2.

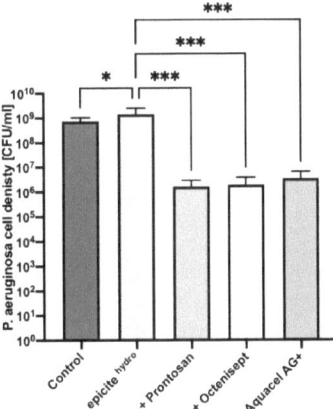

Figure 2. Log_{10} cell density of *P. aeruginosa* (ATCC 700888) 24-hour biofilm following 48-hour treatment with the test dressings. All dressings were tested in triplicate. Error bars represent standard deviation of the mean. Asterisks represent the significant difference between the samples and the untreated control or epicite[hydro]® exclusively.

3.3. 24-Hour CDC Bioreactor Model—C. albicans

After a 24-hour treatment of the *C. albicans* biofilms with unloaded epicite[hydro]® dressings, a fungal density of 2.04×10^6 CFU/mL was observed. In comparison, the untreated biofilm showed a fungal density of 1.45×10^6 CFU/mL. Treatment with unloaded epicite[hydro]® dressings therefore resulted in a slightly higher fungal density with a 0.1 log increase ($p = 0.0317$). In biofilms treated with epicite[hydro]® loaded with Prontosan® or Octenisept® and the positive control Aquacel®Ag Extra, no colonies were observed, exhibiting a 6.2 log reduction in bacterial cell density ($p = 0.0001$). The fungal density reduction of *C. albicans* with all test dressings is displayed in Figure 3.

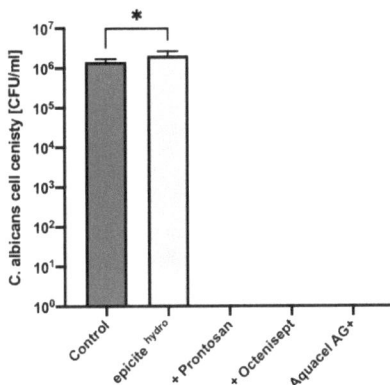

Figure 3. Log_{10} cell density of *C. albicans* (ATCC 10231) 24-h biofilm following 24-h treatment with the test dressings. All dressings were tested in triplicate. Error bars represent standard deviation of the mean. Asterisks represent the significant difference between the samples and the untreated control.

3.4. Effect of Prolonged Antiseptic Treatment In Vivo

To analyze whether the wound healing process would be affected by a prolonged exposure to the antiseptic solutions tested, we performed a 7-day treatment using an in vivo porcine model. During the treatment period, epicite^{hydro}® carrying the antiseptic solutions was left continuously in contact with the wound bed. An example for histological cuts prepared from the regenerated tissues at the end of the treatment can be observed in Figure 4. H&E staining offers the possibility to clearly observe the regenerated tissues, while allowing the observation and quantification of extra parameters, such as the thickness of the BNC dressing and presence of exudate at the wound bed surface. No particular histological difference was observed for the wounds treated with the BNC alone (Figure 4A) compared to the same treatment in combination with Octenisept® (Figure 4B) or with Prontosan® (Figure 4C). The dried aspect of the BNC dressing after 7 days (Figure 5A) indicates that its content was successfully delivered into the wound bed. All the morphometric results obtained from the analyzed tissues were comparable, with no statistical significance being observed. The wound closure rate for the wounds treated with epicite^{hydro}® and with the BNC loaded with Octenisept® or Prontosan® after 7 days (Figure 5B) achieved rates above 75%. Both epidermal average thickness (Figure 5C) and new dermal average thickness (Figure 5D) achieved similar results for all three treatments. The area of exudate present at the last day of treatment was also very similar for all the treatments, with no difference being observed (Figure 5E), indicating that the presence of the antiseptics did not interfere in the exudate production. Despite the BNC dressing being loaded with antiseptics comprising different formulations, in comparison to the original solution present in epicite^{hydro}®, the thickness of the material at the end of the treatment was comparable (Figure 5F). This last result indicates that the evaporation process was not affected.

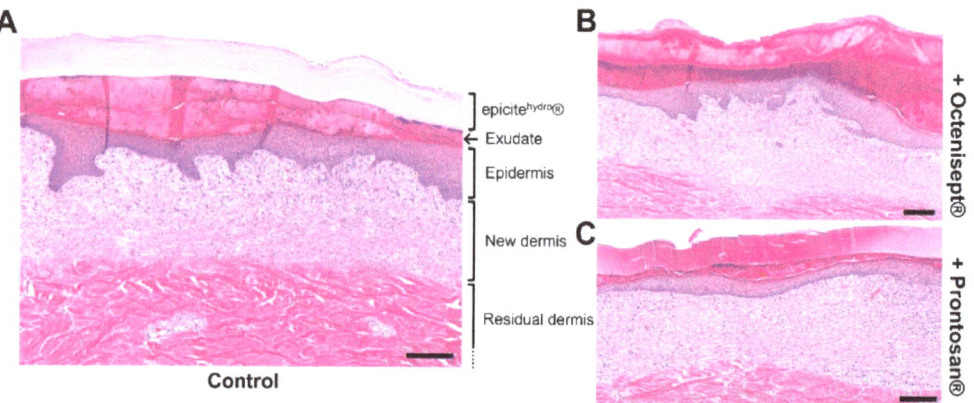

Figure 4. Histological aspects of the regenerated tissue. H&E stainings of representative examples of the regenerated tissue after 7 days of treatment with epicite^{hydro}® (n = 16 wounds) (**A**), epicite^{hydro}® combined with Octenisept® (n = 24 wounds) (**B**) and combined with Prontosan® (n = 24 wounds) (**C**). Scale bars representing 200 µm.

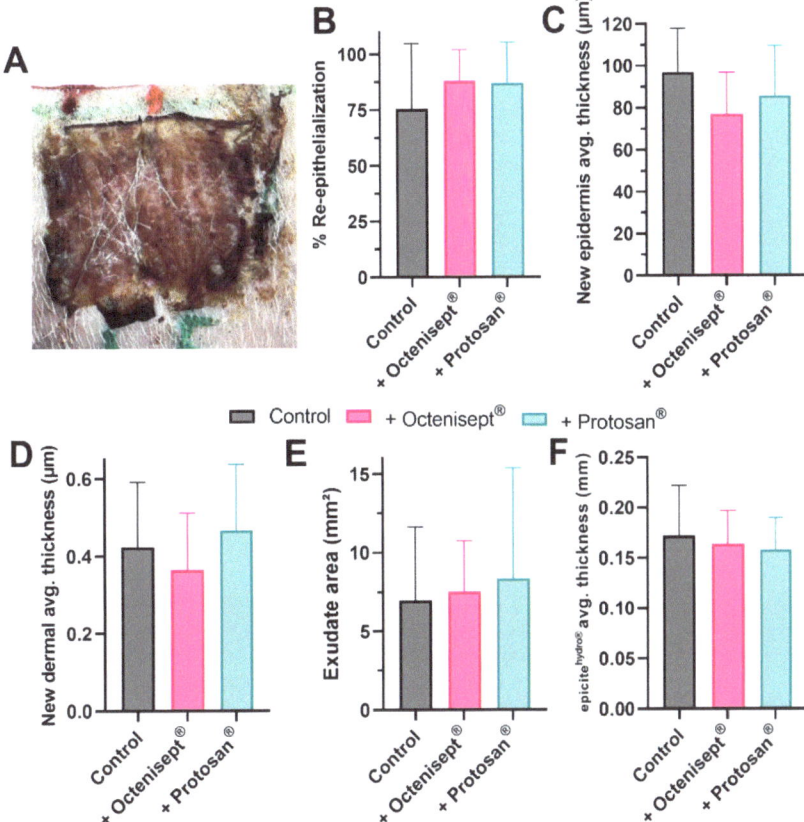

Figure 5. Influence of a 7-day treatment using antiseptics on the wound healing process outcome. Representative image of an epicite^hydro® dressing applied over the wound bed after the 7-day treatment. (**A**). Bar diagrams comprising the results for the percentage of re-epithelialization (**B**), average new epidermal thickness (**C**), average new dermal thickness (**D**), exudate area at day 7 (**E**) and epicite^hydro® dressing average thickness at day 7 (**F**) for the wounds treated using epicite^hydro® alone or combined with Octenisept® or with Prontosan®. The results are presented as mean and standard deviation of the mean.

4. Discussion

Chronic wounds are typically contaminated with pathogenic biofilms causing the prolonging of the inflammatory processes of wound healing, thereby complicating the healing process [14]. The major burden of chronic wounds on patients and healthcare providers has led to extensive research on therapeutic strategies within the past decades [14]. The current standard of care for chronic wounds includes wound swabs, cleaning, dressing and, if necessary, debridement of the wound bed [15].

In addition, environment sensors, using pH, hydration, odor or optical sensors, are available to monitor and manage biofilms and detect early changes in the wound bed associated with pathological wound healing [15]. New strategies of therapeutic intervention may also include the targeting of the wound microenvironment [15].

As another, well-established approach, the dynamic concept of wound bed preparation is particularly beneficial in chronic wounds that fail to progress [16]. This concept comprises comprehensive strategies of tissue management, inflammation and infection control, moisture balance and epithelial advancement (T.I.M.E) to maximize the wound healing potential [16]. However, infection control via targeting and eradicating pathogenic biofilms is especially challenging, since biofilms can be highly tolerant and resistant to antibiotics and antiseptics [2,17].

A variety of molecular mechanisms are thought to contribute to biofilm resistance against antimicrobial agents, which may subsequently lead to treatment failure [2]. Despite the partially limited effect, recent consensus guidelines recommend topical antiseptics as a first-line therapy in the treatment of chronic wounds colonized with a pathogenic biofilm [17].

Prior studies by our research group showed the effective—and clinically feasible—loading and also the release capacity of octenidine- (Octenisept®) and povidone-iodine (Betaisodona®)-based antiseptics in BNC-based wound dressings [11,12]: the antimicrobial efficacy of antiseptic-loaded BNC against *S. aureus* was tested, whereby dose-dependency was shown [11]. In the present study, the antimicrobial activities of BNC loaded with the PHMB-based antiseptic Prontosan® or the octenidine-based antiseptic Octenisept® were tested against a silver-containing dressing showing excellent results in diminishing biofilms.

4.1. Antimicrobial Activity in Gram-Positive Bacteria

Prior in vitro studies by Zmejkosk et al. on a composite hydrogel of BNC and dehydrogenative polymer of coniferyl alcohol have already confirmed our assumptions on an antibacterial activity on *S. aureus* [18]. For a potential use with commercially available antiseptics, we were able to show an effective reduction in cell density after a 24-hour treatment of a *S. aureus* biofilm with unloaded and loaded epicite$^{hydro®}$ dressings in the present project. Treatment with unloaded epicite$^{hydro®}$ dressings resulted in a statistically significant reduction in bacterial density, while biofilms treated with epicite$^{hydro®}$ loaded with Prontosan® resulted in a 4.9 log reduction. Loading with Octenisept® even resulted in a complete eradication of the colony, similar to the treatment with the silver-containing dressing control Aquacel®Ag Extra.

Other in vitro studies have already demonstrated the efficacy of PHMB-based antiseptics on Gram-positive bacteria [19]; however, a slower onset of antimicrobial activity compared to other formulations is noted [20]. Furthermore, conflicting evidence regarding the antimicrobial activity of PHMB-based antiseptics was raised [21]. These findings may explain the reduced antimicrobial effect of Prontosan® compared to Octenisept® or silver-based dressings. Future studies evaluating a prolonged treatment period are of utmost importance to elucidate the full potential of each antiseptic solution.

In comparison to BNC loaded with PHMB-based antiseptics, complete biofilm eradication was feasible within a 24-hour treatment with Octenisept®-loaded BNC or a silver-based dressing. Although silver has been positioned among first-line options for wound infection and is recommended for the treatment of pathogenic biofilms [2], bacterial resistance is well documented [22,23]. In contrast, no reports of bacterial resistance on octenidine exist to our knowledge. A recent in -vitro study by Günther et al. even demonstrated a great level of bacterial metabolic inhibition by octenidine-based antiseptics in a biofilm of methicillin-resistant *S. aureus* [24]. Based on these findings, treatment with octenidine-based antiseptics such as with Octenisept® may be preferable to other options, even in biofilms of drug-resistant Gram-positive bacteria.

4.2. Antimicrobial Activity in Gram-Negative Bacteria

Cell density of a 48-hour *P. aeruginosa* biofilm treated with unloaded epicite$^{hydro®}$ exclusively slightly increased after a treatment period of 24 h. However, if loaded with Prontosan® or Octenisept®, 2.7 log and 2.6 log reductions in biofilm cell density were found compared to the unloaded epicite$^{hydro®}$. A similar log reduction was achieved in the positive control.

Bacterial resistance against silver is rare, but it has been documented in Gram-negative bacteria including *P. aeruginosa* [25]. Contrary to this, no reports of bacterial resistance have been documented for PHMB-based antiseptics [2], which were showing the best results in the present project. A variety of studies proved the initial antibacterial effect of silver-based wound dressings on (even multi-drug resistant) *P. aeruginosa* [26,27]; however, bacterial tolerance against silver may develop over time when biofilms are evident. This mechanism may explain the initial therapeutic success also observed in our in vitro experiments. Despite a possible silver release of dressings such as Aquacel®Ag Extra being reported for up to two weeks [28], the potential long-term limits of silver-based dressings in chronic wounds compared to antiseptic-loaded BNC dressings are yet to be elucidated.

4.3. Antimicrobial Activity in Fungi

Treatment of a *C. albicans* biofilm with unloaded epicite$^{hydro®}$ dressings resulted in a slightly higher fungal cell density. However, if loaded with Prontosan® or Octenisept®, colonies were completely eradicated. Treatment with Aquacel®Ag Extra resulted in a complete eradication as well. While studies on the efficacy of PHMB-based antiseptics in *C. albicans* infections with a high organic load are lacking, significant results for octenidine-based antiseptics have recently been published by Spettel et al. [29]. The authors reported a full antimicrobial effect for *C. albicans* and other Candida strains after a contact time of only 30 s. Therefore, octenidine-based antiseptics may be preferable in fungal colonization when it comes to a routine clinical use. The combination with BNC-based dressings may be beneficial to generate a prolonged and steady concentration release of active ingredients.

Since fungi can sense suitable ambient pH for adhesion, growth and invasion, pH monitoring of a wound may be an effective approach in the prevention of colonization [30]. Especially, diabetic patients (with diabetic foot ulcers) expressing a higher pH in intertriginous areas are at risk to candidiasis, mostly with *C. albicans* [30]. After initial colonization, fungi are further increasing pH of the wound bed, resulting in a clinically manifest infection [30]. In addition to an antiseptic enhancement of BNC, pH monitoring in a sterile and easy-to-handle setting is possible [9]. When chemically functionalized with indicator dye, pH monitoring through BNC can be performed without the removal of the dressing or wound contact of a pH monitor device [9]. Potential combinations of these features in future "smart dressings" may enable a release of active substances only above a certain pH-value. Epicite$^{hydro®}$ as an advanced wound dressing might therefore not only assist in the treatment of pathogenic biofilms, but as well in its prevention, ultimately reducing the burden of chronic wounds.

4.4. General Assumptions on the Use of Silver-Based Dressings vs. Antiseptic-Loaded BNC

Several differences of topical antiseptics regarding anti-biofilm efficacy, safety, and tolerability in chronic wounds have been reported [2]. The available silver-based dressings commonly used in a variety of applications due to antibacterial properties not only differ in their construction and their chemical composition of the active layer, but also in their silver forms [31]. A recent study revealed that the amount of silver contained in a dressing is often not stated by the manufacturer [31]. The authors show a potential DNA-damage of silver, released via dressings and diffused into intact porcine dermis [31]. Potential silver toxicity due to the unawareness of the amount released can therefore be detrimental to proliferating cells in already healing wounds, supporting recommendations that silver-based dressings should only be applied to highly infected, chronic wounds [31].

In comparison, BNC-based wound dressings can be used for a variety of applications (e.g., [10]) and have been shown to be nontoxic, to provide rapid tissue regeneration as well as capillary formation in the wound area [18]. As previously shown by our group, BNC can additionally be used as an effective carrier of antiseptic solutions, enabling an application in the prevention and treatment of colonized, chronic wounds [11].

4.5. Wound Healing Process in a Prolonged Antiseptic Treatment Period

Cell survival in vitro was already reported to be affected by various antiseptic molecules, including PHMB- and octenidine-based solutions [32]. On the other hand, reduced cytotoxicity and interesting biocompatibility indexes were observed for the same antiseptics when applied in specific concentrations [33]. The detrimental effect of the antiseptics on the viability of cells, such as fibroblasts and keratinocytes, seems to be higher in vitro when tested on isolated cells, than in a more complex system [34]. Usually, the tests are conducted exposing the cells to short periods of time (a few minutes or a couple of hours) [32,33,35,36]. To our knowledge, so far, no test has been performed for longer incubation periods nor utilizing an in vivo model to analyze how the healing processes are affected. Since the potential application against pathogens capable of producing biofilms here proposed used a 24 h treatment, we decided to analyze how the wound healing process in vivo would be affected by a continuous exposure of the antiseptics. In previous works, we were able to report a sustained delivery in vitro of the antiseptic solutions over 48 h using the BNC as a delivery platform [11,12]. In our in vivo tests, we decided to use a 7-day treatment, to guarantee that the integral BNC content would be delivered and to assess the influence of the antiseptics over a prolonged period. No significant difference was observed for all the healing parameters analyzed. Both epidermal and dermal regeneration results were comparable with the control. Wound closure rates, for instance, achieved results above 75% for all treatments, which are in line with recent reports [37]. Additionally, results for the exudate area indicate that physiological secretion was not disturbed by the presence of the antiseptics. Considering the physicochemical aspects of the BNC dressing combined with the antiseptics, the comparable results for the average thickness of the dressing at the end of the treatment suggest that the evaporation process was not impaired nor promoted. This result is important, to show that the moisture offered by the dressing remains constant even after the combination with antiseptics. An ideal moisture balance was already reported as being crucial to support the healing process [38–41]. These results confirm that the method here proposed to treat pathogens capable of producing biofilm would not negatively influence the wound healing process.

Nevertheless, eradication of pathogenic biofilms and reduction of the burden caused by chronic wounds may not be feasible via this approach exclusively. To achieve wound healing, addressing other factors regarding the patient's general health or the wound's physical environment is of utmost importance [42].

In addition to the delivery of antibiotics, physical treatment approaches such as hyperbaric oxygen therapy, low-level laser therapy and electrical stimulation can be used in specific cases to accelerate the healing of chronic ulcers, although inconsistent success is reported [43]. Negative pressure wound therapy is a different physical treatment approach indicated for deep chronic and very exudating wounds, based on differential suction or vacuum creation onto the wound bed to enhance fluid removal, reduce edema and alter the wound microenvironment for subsequently performing skin grafting [44]. An analysis of 11 trials by Wynn et al. showed a significant reduction of the wound surface area through negative pressure wound therapy [45], which might as well be feasible via the use of advanced dressings, e.g., polylactide wound dressings [46]. To our understanding, a holistic assessment of the patient and the wound is essential to choose the optimal strategy out of multiple to prevent or treat chronic wounds and optimally manage patients.

4.6. Limitations

All biofilm experiments were performed in vitro, although tested antiseptics, BNC-based and silver-based wound dressings are already available on the market. The results of the release experiments of the antiseptics may not be directly transferred into clinical practice without consideration. Since pathogenic biofilms may consist of an individual mix of bacteria and fungi, the use of agar plates is not a comparable receiving medium to an actual *clinical* wound bed. Furthermore, the interaction of exudate occurring in a (chronic) wound with BNC as well as the antiseptic solution cannot be assessed within this setting. To confirm a superior antimicrobial efficacy of the loaded BNC-based wound dressings compared to commercially available (silver-based) dressings, further clinical studies are necessary. In vivo experiments were conducted in a porcine model; however this model is already widely accepted for preclinical experiments [47]. Ultimately, there is a great demand for prevention and treatment strategies for chronic wounds, and valuable results could be retrieved from this study.

5. Conclusions

Available evidence suggests that the majority of chronic wounds are colonized by pathogenic biofilms hindering wound healing, resulting in ineffective treatment, burdening both the patient and the healthcare providers. BNC-based wound dressings loaded with commercially available antiseptics demonstrate a potent efficacy against biofilms formed by a variety of microbes found to be prevalent within chronic wounds, including *S aureus*, *P. aeruginosa*, and *C. albicans*. Additionally, no negative influence was observed in the wound healing parameters analyzed, showing that even a 7-day treatment using the BNC loaded with antiseptics would not disturb the normal healing process. Results are comparable to available silver-based wound dressings, whereby further advantages of BNC such as the possibility for pH-monitoring of the wound bed are to be highlighted. Antiseptic-loaded BNC-based wound dressings might therefore be an effective modality in the prevention and treatment of colonized, chronic wounds. Future studies are essential to investigate and compare the in vivo efficacy of this approach in clinical care.

Author Contributions: H.L. and I.B.d.M. conceived the study and designed the trial. M.F. and L.-P.K. supervised the conduct of the trial and data collection. H.L., S.P.N. and A.C.T. managed the data, including quality control. I.B.d.M. chaired the data oversight committee. H.L. drafted the manuscript, and all authors contributed substantially to its revision. M.F. and L.-P.K. were responsible for the paper as a whole. All authors have read and agreed to the published version of the manuscript.

Funding: This research received no external funding.

Institutional Review Board Statement: The animal study protocol was approved by the Animal Care and Use Committee (Veterinary University Vienna, Austrian Ministry of Science and Research) (protocol code GZ 2020-0.701.443, 4 December 2020).

Informed Consent Statement: Not applicable.

Data Availability Statement: All data generated or analyzed during this study are included in this published article.

Conflicts of Interest: The authors declare no conflict of interest. Epicite^{hydro}® wound dressings were provided by QRSKIN GmbH (Würzburg, Germany) free of charge. QRSKIN GmbH did not influence the structure or content of this study in any way. The study was conducted at the 5D Health Protection Group Ltd., Centre of Excellence in Biofilm Science Liverpool, United Kingdom. There has been no significant financial support for this work that could have influenced its outcome.

References

1. Guo, S.; DiPietro, L.A. Factors affecting wound healing. *J. Dent. Res.* **2010**, *89*, 219–229. [CrossRef]
2. Alves, P.J.; Barreto, R.T.; Barrois, B.M.; Gryson, L.G.; Meaume, S.; Monstrey, S.J. Update on the role of antiseptics in the management of chronic wounds with critical colonisation and/or biofilm. *Int. Wound J.* **2021**, *18*, 342–358. [CrossRef] [PubMed]
3. White, R.J.; Cutting, K.F. Critical colonization—The concept under scrutiny. *Ostomy. Wound. Manag.* **2006**, *52*, 50–56.
4. Wilson, C.; Lukowicz, R.; Merchant, S.; Valquier-Flynn, H.; Caballero, J.; Sandoval, J.; Okuom, M.; Huber, C.; Brooks, T.D.; Wilson, E.; et al. Quantitative and qualitative assessment methods for biofilm growth: A mini-review. *Res. Rev. J. Eng. Technol.* **2017**, *6*, 4. Available online: http://www.ncbi.nlm.nih.gov/pubmed/30214915 (accessed on 18 August 2022).
5. Malone, M.; Bjarnsholt, T.; McBain, A.J.; James, G.A.; Stoodley, P.; Leaper, D.; Tachi, M.; Schultz, G.; Swanson, T.; Wolcott, R.D. The prevalence of biofilms in chronic wounds: A systematic review and meta-analysis of published data. *J. Wound Care* **2017**, *26*, 20–25. [CrossRef] [PubMed]
6. Kadam, S.; Shai, S.; Shahane, A.; Kaushik, K.S. Recent advances in non-conventional antimicrobial approaches for chronic wound biofilms: Have we found the 'chink in the armor'? *Biomedicines* **2019**, *7*, 35. [CrossRef]
7. Percival, S.L.; Vuotto, C.; Donelli, G.; Lipsky, B.A. Biofilms and wounds: An identification algorithm and potential treatment options. *Adv. Wound Care* **2015**, *4*, 389–397. [CrossRef]
8. Pomares, G.; Huguet, S.; Dap, F.; Dautel, G. Contaminated wounds: Effectiveness of debridement for reducing bacterial load. *Hand Surg. Rehabil.* **2016**, *35*, 266–270. [CrossRef]

9. Nischwitz, S.; de Mattos, I.B.; Hofmann, E.; Groeber-Becker, F.; Funk, M.; Mohr, G.; Branski, L.; Mautner, S.; Kamolz, L. Continuous pH monitoring in wounds using a composite indicator dressing—A feasibility study. *Burns* **2019**, *45*, 1336–1341. [CrossRef]
10. Holzer, J.C.; Tiffner, K.; Kainz, S.; Reisenegger, P.; de Mattos, I.B.; Funk, M.; Lemarchand, T.; Laaff, H.; Bal, A.; Birngruber, T.; et al. A novel human ex-vivo burn model and the local cooling effect of a bacterial nanocellulose-based wound dressing. *Burns* **2020**, *46*, 1924–1932. [CrossRef]
11. de Mattos, I.B.; Nischwitz, S.P.; Tuca, A.-C.; Groeber-Becker, F.; Funk, M.; Birngruber, T.; Mautner, S.I.; Kamolz, L.-P.; Holzer, J.C. Delivery of antiseptic solutions by a bacterial cellulose wound dressing: Uptake, release and antibacterial efficacy of octenidine and povidone-iodine. *Burns* **2020**, *46*, 918–927. [CrossRef] [PubMed]
12. de Mattos, I.B.; Holzer, J.C.; Tuca, A.-C.; Groeber-Becker, F.; Funk, M.; Popp, D.; Mautner, S.; Birngruber, T.; Kamolz, L.-P. Uptake of PHMB in a bacterial nanocellulose-based wound dressing: A feasible clinical procedure. *Burns* **2019**, *45*, 898–904. [CrossRef] [PubMed]
13. Ip, M.; Lui, S.L.; Poon, V.K.M.; Lung, I.; Burd, A. Antimicrobial activities of silver dressings: An in vitro comparison. *J. Med. Microbiol.* **2006**, *55*, 59–63. [CrossRef] [PubMed]
14. Raziyeva, K.; Kim, Y.; Zharkinbekov, Z.; Kassymbek, K.; Jimi, S.; Saparov, A. Immunology of acute and chronic wound healing. *Biomolecules* **2021**, *11*, 700. [CrossRef] [PubMed]
15. Dreifke, M.B.; Jayasuriya, A.A.; Jayasuriya, A.C. Current wound healing procedures and potential care. *Mater. Sci. Eng. C* **2015**, *48*, 651–662. [CrossRef]
16. Halim, A.S.; Khoo, T.L.; Saad, A.Z.M. Wound bed preparation from a clinical perspective. *Indian J. Plast. Surg.* **2012**, *45*, 193–202. [CrossRef]
17. Schultz, G.; Bjarnsholt, T.; James, G.A.; Leaper, D.J.; McBain, A.J.; Malone, M.; Stoodley, P.; Swanson, T.; Tachi, M.; Wolcott, R.D.; et al. Consensus guidelines for the identification and treatment of biofilms in chronic nonhealing wounds. *Wound Repair Regen.* **2017**, *25*, 744–757. [CrossRef]
18. Zmejkoski, D.; Spasojević, D.; Orlovska, I.; Kozyrovska, N.; Soković, M.; Glamočlija, J.; Dmitrović, S.; Matović, B.; Tasić, N.; Maksimović, V.; et al. Bacterial cellulose-lignin composite hydrogel as a promising agent in chronic wound healing. *Int. J. Biol. Macromol.* **2018**, *118*, 494–503. [CrossRef]
19. Fjeld, H.; Lingaas, E. Polyheksanid-sikkerhet og effekt som antiseptikum. *Tidsskr. Den Nor. Legeforening* **2016**, *136*, 707–711. [CrossRef]
20. Koburger, T.; Hubner, N.-O.; Braun, M.; Siebert, J.; Kramer, A. Standardized comparison of antiseptic efficacy of triclosan, PVP-iodine, octenidine dihydrochloride, polyhexanide and chlorhexidine digluconate. *J. Antimicrob. Chemother.* **2010**, *65*, 1712–1719. [CrossRef]
21. Kamaruzzaman, N.F.; Chong, S.Q.Y.; Edmondson-Brown, K.M.; Ntow-Boahene, W.; Bardiau, M.; Good, L. Bactericidal and anti-biofilm effects of polyhexamethylene biguanide in models of intracellular and biofilm of staphylococcus aureus isolated from bovine mastitis. *Front. Microbiol.* **2017**, *8*, 1518. [CrossRef] [PubMed]
22. Panáček, A.; Kvítek, L.; Smékalová, M.; Večeřová, R.; Kolář, M.; Röderová, M.; Dyčka, F.; Šebela, M.; Prucek, R.; Tomanec, O.; et al. Bacterial resistance to silver nanoparticles and how to overcome it. *Nat. Nanotechnol.* **2017**, *13*, 65–71. [CrossRef]
23. Finley, P.J.; Norton, R.; Austin, C.; Mitchell, A.; Zank, S.; Durham, P. Unprecedented silver resistance in clinically isolated enterobacteriaceae: Major implications for burn and wound management. *Antimicrob. Agents Chemother.* **2015**, *59*, 4734–4741. [CrossRef]
24. Günther, F.; Blessing, B.; Dapunt, U.; Mischnik, A.; Mutters, N.T. Ability of chlorhexidine, octenidine, polyhexanide and chloroxylenol to inhibit metabolism of biofilm-forming clinical multidrug-resistant organisms. *J. Infect. Prev.* **2021**, *22*, 12–18. [CrossRef] [PubMed]
25. Randall, C.P.; Gupta, A.; Jackson, N.; Busse, D.; O'Neill, A.J. Silver resistance in Gram-negative bacteria: A dissection of endogenous and exogenous mechanisms. *J. Antimicrob. Chemother.* **2015**, *70*, 1037–1046. [CrossRef] [PubMed]
26. Percival, S.L.; Bowler, P.; Woods, E.J. Assessing the effect of an antimicrobial wound dressing on biofilms. *Wound Repair Regen.* **2008**, *16*, 52–57. [CrossRef]
27. Liao, S.; Zhang, Y.; Pan, X.; Zhu, F.; Jiang, C.; Liu, Q.; Cheng, Z.; Dai, G.; Wu, G.; Wang, L.; et al. Antibacterial activity and mechanism of silver nanoparticles against multidrug-resistant *Pseudomonas aeruginosa*. *Int. J. Nanomed.* **2019**, *14*, 1469–1487. [CrossRef]
28. Caruso, D.M.; Foster, K.N.; Hermans, M.H.E.; Rick, C. Aquacel Ag® in the management of partial-thickness burns: Results of a clinical trial. *J. Burn Care Rehabil.* **2004**, *25*, 89–97. [CrossRef]
29. Spettel, K.; Bumberger, D.; Camp, I.; Kriz, R.; Willinger, B. Efficacy of octenidine against emerging echinocandin-, azole- and multidrug-resistant *Candida albicans* and *Candida glabrata*. *J. Glob. Antimicrob. Resist.* **2022**, *29*, 23–28. [CrossRef]
30. Rippke, F.; Berardesca, E.; Weber, T.M. pH and microbial infections. *pH Ski. Issues Chall.* **2018**, *54*, 87–94.
31. Nešporová, K.; Pavlík, V.; Šafránková, B.; Vágnerová, H.; Odrášková, P.; Žídek, O.; Císařová, N.; Skoroplyas, S.; Kubala, L.; Velebný, V. Effects of wound dressings containing silver on skin and immune cells. *Sci. Rep.* **2020**, *10*, 15216. [CrossRef]
32. van Meurs, S.J.; Gawlitta, D.; Heemstra, K.A.; Poolman, R.W.; Vogely, H.C.; Kruyt, M.C. Selection of an optimal antiseptic solution for intraoperative irrigation. *J. Bone Jt. Surg.* **2014**, *96*, 285–291. [CrossRef] [PubMed]
33. Muller, G.; Kramer, A. Biocompatibility index of antiseptic agents by parallel assessment of antimicrobial activity and cellular cytotoxicity. *J. Antimicrob. Chemother.* **2008**, *61*, 1281–1287. [CrossRef] [PubMed]

34. Bigliardi, P.L.; Alsagoff, S.A.L.; El-Kafrawi, H.Y.; Pyon, J.-K.; Wa, C.T.C.; Villa, M.A. Povidone iodine in wound healing: A review of current concepts and practices. *Int. J. Surg.* **2017**, *44*, 260–268. [CrossRef]
35. Thongrueang, N.; Liu, S.-S.; Hsu, H.-Y.; Lee, H.-H. An in vitro comparison of antimicrobial efficacy and cytotoxicity between povidone-iodine and chlorhexidine for treating clinical endometritis in dairy cows. *PLoS ONE* **2022**, *17*, e0271274. [CrossRef]
36. Chindera, K.; Mahato, M.; Sharma, A.K.; Horsley, H.; Kloc-Muniak, K.; Kamaruzzaman, N.F.; Kumar, S.; McFarlane, A.; Stach, J.; Bentin, T.; et al. The antimicrobial polymer PHMB enters cells and selectively condenses bacterial chromosomes. *Sci. Rep.* **2016**, *6*, 23121. [CrossRef] [PubMed]
37. Tuca, A.-C.; de Mattos, I.B.; Funk, M.; Winter, R.; Palackic, A.; Groeber-Becker, F.; Kruse, D.; Kukla, F.; Lemarchand, T.; Kamolz, L.-P. Orchestrating the dermal/epidermal tissue ratio during wound healing by controlling the moisture content. *Biomedicines* **2022**, *10*, 1286. [CrossRef]
38. Winter, G.D. Formation of the scab and the rate of epithelization of superficial wounds in the skin of the young domestic pig. *Nature* **1962**, *193*, 293–294. [CrossRef]
39. Winter, G.D.; Scales, J.T. Effect of air drying and dressings on the surface of a wound. *Nature* **1963**, *197*, 91–99. [CrossRef]
40. Bishop, S.M.; Walker, M.; Rogers, A.A.; Chen, W.Y.J. Importance of moisture balance at the wound-dressing interface. *J. Wound Care* **2003**, *12*, 125–128. [CrossRef]
41. Okan, D.; Woo, K.; Ayello, E.A.; Sibbald, G. The role of moisture balance in wound healing. *Adv. Ski. Wound Care* **2007**, *20*, 39–53. [CrossRef]
42. Daeschlein, G. Antimicrobial and antiseptic strategies in wound management. *Int. Wound J.* **2013**, *10*, 9–14. [CrossRef] [PubMed]
43. Omar, M.T.; Gwada, R.F.; Shaheen, A.A.; Saggini, R. Extracorporeal shockwave therapy for the treatment of chronic wound of lower extremity: Current perspective and systematic review. *Int. Wound J.* **2017**, *14*, 898–908. [CrossRef]
44. Takagi, S.; Oyama, T.; Jimi, S.; Saparov, A.; Ohjimi, H. A novel autologous micrografts technology in combination with negative pressure wound therapy (NPWT) for quick granulation tissue formation in chronic/refractory ulcer. *Healthcare* **2020**, *8*, 513. [CrossRef] [PubMed]
45. Wynn, M.; Freeman, S. The efficacy of negative pressure wound therapy for diabetic foot ulcers: A systematised review. *J. Tissue Viability* **2019**, *28*, 152–160. [CrossRef]
46. Nischwitz, S.P.; Popp, D.; Shubitidze, D.; Luze, H.; Zrim, R.; Klemm, K.; Rapp, M.; Haller, H.L.; Feisst, M.; Kamolz, L. The successful use of polylactide wound dressings for chronic lower leg wounds: A retrospective analysis. *Int. Wound J.* **2021**, *19*, 1180–1187. [CrossRef] [PubMed]
47. Parnell, L.K.S.; Volk, S.W. The evolution of animal models in wound healing research: 1993–2017. *Adv. Wound Care* **2019**, *8*, 692–702. [CrossRef]

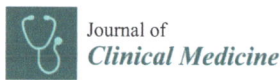

Review

Locoregional Flaps for the Reconstruction of Midface Skin Defects: A Collection of Key Surgical Techniques

Giovanni Salzano [1,*], Francesco Maffia [1], Luigi Angelo Vaira [2,3], Umberto Committeri [1], Chiara Copelli [4], Fabio Maglitto [4], Alfonso Manfuso [4], Vincenzo Abbate [1], Paola Bonavolontà [1], Alfonso Scarpa [5], Luigi Califano [1] and Giovanni Dell'Aversana Orabona [1]

1 Maxillofacial Surgery Operative Unit, Department of Neurosciences, Reproductive and Odontostomatological Sciences, Federico II University of Naples, 80131 Naples, Italy; francesco.maffia@gmail.com (F.M.); umbertocommitteri@gmail.com (U.C.); vincenzo.abbate@unina.it (V.A.); paola.bonavolonta@unina.it (P.B.); califano@unina.it (L.C.); giovanni.dellaversanaorabona@unina.it (G.D.O.)
2 Maxillofacial Surgery Operative Unit, Department of Medicine, Surgery and Pharmacy, University of Sassari, 07100 Sassari, Italy; lavaira@uniss.it
3 Biomedical Science Department, PhD School of Biomedical Science, University of Sassari, 07100 Sassari, Italy
4 Maxillofacial Surgery Operative Unit, Department of Interdisciplinary Medicine, Aldo Moro University of Bari, 70120 Bari, Italy; chiara.copelli@uniba.it (C.C.); fabio.maglitto@policlinico.ba.it (F.M.); alfonso.manfuso@policlinico.ba.it (A.M.)
5 Department of Medicine and Surgery, University of Salerno, 84081 Salerno, Italy; alfonsoscarpa@yahoo.it
* Correspondence: giovannisalzanomd@gmail.com

Abstract: Background: The reconstruction of midface skin defects represents a challenge for the head and neck surgeon due to the midface's significant role in defining important facial traits. Due to the high complexity of the midface region, there is no possibility to use one definitive flap for all purposes. For moderate defects, the most common reconstructive techniques are represented by regional flaps. These flaps can be defined as donor tissue with a pedunculated axial blood supply not necessarily adjacent to the defect. The aim of this study is to highlight the more common surgical techniques adopted for midface reconstruction, providing a focus on each technique with its description and indications. Methods: A literature review was conducted using PubMed, an international database. The target of the research was to collect at least 10 different surgical techniques. Results: Twelve different techniques were selected and cataloged. The flaps included were the bilobed flap, rhomboid flap, facial-artery-based flaps (nasolabial flap, island composite nasal flap, retroangular flap), cervicofacial flap, paramedian forehead flap, frontal hairline island flap, keystone flap, Karapandzic flap, Abbè flap, and Mustardè flap. Conclusions: The study of the facial subunits, the location and size of the defect, the choice of the appropriate flap, and respect for the vascular pedicles are the key elements for optimal outcomes.

Keywords: head and neck reconstruction; midface skin defects; midface locoregional flaps; pedunculated flaps

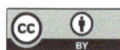

1. Introduction

The reconstruction of midface skin defects represents a challenge for the head and neck surgeon due to its renowned role in defining important facial traits [1]. Midfacial skin defects can originate from neoplasm asportation or be secondary to facial trauma [2]. The term "midface" refers to several anatomical sub-regions including the infraorbital region, malar region, and nasolabial region [3]. The division of the face into facial aesthetic subunits represents a valid method to delimitate the face in regions with similar characteristics [4]. A particularity of these areas is represented by how they show different thicknesses and layers, even among contiguous regions, complicating reconstruction planning [5,6]. Indeed, the functionality and high aesthetical consideration of the midface require the surgeon to find innovative solutions to restore form and function [7]. In the surgical treatment of midface skin defects, a meticulous preoperative assessment is required to properly assess the anticipated gap and to determine the proper reconstructive plan [3]. Split-thickness skin grafts, full-thickness skin grafts, pedunculated flaps, and free flaps are the main surgical options in soft tissue defect reconstruction [8]. Due to the high complexity of the midface region, there is no possibility to use one definitive flap for all purposes, so expanding our surgical arsenal is necessary to overcome reconstruction difficulties [2]. For moderate defects, the most common reconstructive techniques are represented by regional flaps. These flaps can be defined as donor tissue with a pedunculated axial blood supply not necessarily adjacent to the defect [1]. To date, there is no consensus on the most appropriate flap design for specific defects, especially in defects located across more midfacial subunits [9]. The most common pedicle in many of the flaps for midface reconstruction is represented by the facial artery: thanks to its course and its collateral branches, it allows almost complete coverage of the whole region [10]. The choice of locoregional flaps is also supported by favorable skin color- and texture-match characteristics [11]. The continuous development of surgical techniques has led to a wide armamentarium of different midfacial regional flaps, related to high facial vascularization [12]. The aim of this study is to highlight the more common surgical techniques adopted for the reconstruction of a complex area such as the midface. The authors provide a focus on each technique with its description and indications based on defect size.

2. Materials and Methods

2.1. Literature Review

Initial background research was conducted to outline the conceptual foundations of the study: the reconstruction of midface soft tissue. A literature review was conducted using PubMed, an international database. The keywords used were: "head and neck surgery", "head and neck reconstruction", "head and neck skin defects", and "midface skin defects". The database used was screened using the keywords in combination with "surgical flaps", and "locoregional flaps" included in the research string.

2.2. Study Selection

The review of the literature was conducted in November 2022. The researchers decided to not include a chronological limit to the research. The target of the research was to collect at least 10 different surgical techniques with diverse complexity indexes. Adopted inclusion criteria were (a) articles written in English; (b) technique studies, retrospective studies, and prospective studies; (c) studies describing the surgical reconstruction of a midface skin defect; and (d) the adoption of pedunculated flaps harvested with only soft tissue. Exclusion criteria were (a) articles not describing the surgical technique adopted; (b) articles involving more complex or multilayered defects; and (c) the adoption of free flaps. The studies matching the inclusion criteria were recognized and were read in full to perform the data extraction.

2.3. Surgical Techniques Data Extraction

After individuating the different techniques, data were extracted accounting for complete technique explanations, descriptions of application areas, and descriptions of the defect's diameter. When the same technique was reported in more than one study, the most precise was preferred and selected. All data were stored in a digital database including the technique name, the type of the adopted flap, the main midface region treated, suggested secondary regions, and skin defect size (small, medium, large). The classification in sizes followed a centimetric division found in the literature: 1.5–2 cm for "small", 2–3 cm for "medium", and >3 cm for "large". Additional or missing information was compared among similar studies and collected in the digital database.

3. Results

Among the studies obtained, 12 different techniques were selected and cataloged. The main characteristics of each technique are reported in Table 1.

Table 1. Main characteristics of each technique in alphabetical order, divided by type of flap, main midface region, secondary regions, and skin defect size.

Technique Adopted	Type of Flap	Main Midface Region	Secondary Regions	Skin Defect Size
Abbè Flap	Rotational Flap	Upper Lip	-	Small–Medium
Bilobed Flap	Transpositional Flap	Nose	Eyelids	Small
Cervicofacial Flap	Rotational/Advancement Flap	Cheek	Periorbital Region, Preauricular, Neck	Large
Frontal Hairline Island Flap	Transpositional Flap	Nose	Canthal, Upper lip	Medium
Island Composite Nasal Flap	Transpositional Flap	Nose (Higher Portion)	-	Medium
Karapandzic Flap	Rotational Flap	Upper lip	Lower Lip	Medium–Large
Keystone Flap	Advancement Flap	Cheek	Nose, Upper Lip	Medium
Mustardè Flap	Rotational Flap	Cheek	Lateral Nose Wall, Lower Eyelid	Medium–Large
Nasolabial Flap	Advancement Flap	Nose	Periorbital Region, Cheek, Upper Lip	Medium
Paramedian Flap	Rotational Flap	Nose	-	Medium–Large
Retroangular Flap	Transpositional Flap	Cheek	Nose, Periorbital Region, Glabella	Medium
Rhomboidal Flap	Transpositional Flap	Cheek	Scalp, Neck, Nose, Eyelids	Medium

The type of flap was divided into transpositional (5/12, 41%), rotational (4/12, 33%), and advancement flaps (2/12 16%). Just one flap was considered both rotational and advancement. The cheek and nose areas were the most described regions (both 5/12, 41%), followed by the upper lip area (2/12, 16%). Defect size indications were mostly "medium" (9/12, 75%).

Surgical Techniques Collection

The highlights of the techniques included are described in the following list:

1. *Bilobed flap*: the bilobed flap (BF) is a single pedicle random pattern cutaneous transposition flap composed of two lobes. Its applications are various, including the hand, scalp, foot, and eyelids, but its main adoption is in nasal reconstruction for its excellent color and texture match with adjacent skin. The BF is used for small nasal defects (1.5 cm). Nasal ala defects are approached with a medially based flap, while tip defects are approached with a laterally based one. The surgical technique requires precise measurements: the first measure is the diameter of the defect (D), then the pivot point is placed at least 0.5 D from the defect; from the pivot point, the outer flap edge is obtained by rotating a suture around the pivot point; an inner arch is marked 0.5 D inside the outer arch; and the first lobe is demarcated with a diameter equal to D, while the second lobe is marked with a width 0.5 higher than D (Figure 1). The dissection is performed above the periosteum and perichondrium. The first lobe covers the excision gap and the second lobe will replace the first lobe, while the gap of the second lobe is closed by direct suture [11].

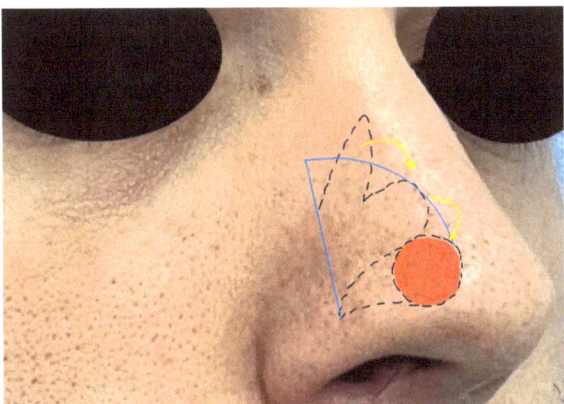

Figure 1. The bilobed flap with its geometrical drawing. Red zone indicate the skin defect, dotted lines indicate cuts, blue lines are geometric landmarks, and yellow arrows indicate flap shifts.

2. *Rhomboid flap*: the rhomboid flap (RF), also known as the Limberg flap, is a transposing rhomboid-shaped flap, used typically for medium-sized defects of the cheek (2–2.5 cm). It can be designed in every direction. The main advantage is that, being adjacent to the defect, it matches the skin color and texture. Its plan is geometrical: the defect is surrounded by a rhomboid with 60° and 120° angles; then, the flap is designed on the short axis (120°), as shown in Figure 2. The Dufourmentel flap is a modification of the Limberg flap and uses angles from 60° to 90° [11,13,14].

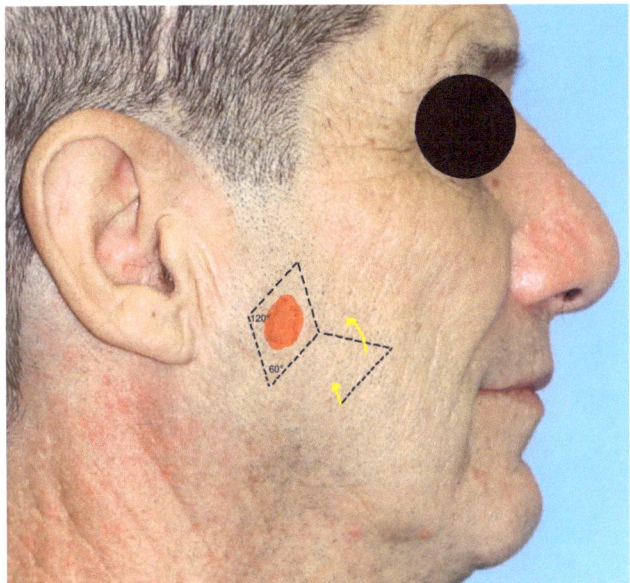

Figure 2. Rhomboid flap with angles and incision lines.

3. Facial-artery-based flaps: The *nasolabial flap (NLF)* is the most adopted advancement flap in the reconstruction of the nasal side wall and ala defects and also cheek and upper lip regions. The NLF is used to cover medium defects close to the flap. It is based on the branches of the facial artery, most commonly on the angular artery. It is

triangular-shaped, with the base of the triangle direct to the defect, while the apex is directed toward the pedicle. Once the flap is mobilized, the surgical wound is closed in a V-Y fashion [2,15] (Figure 3A).

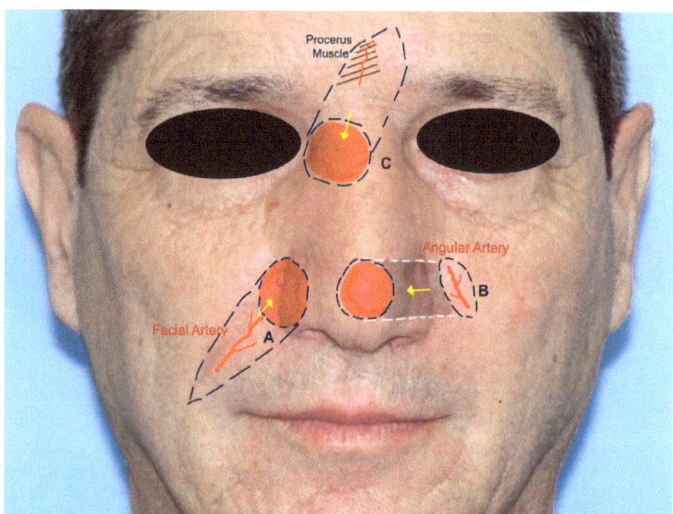

Figure 3. Facial-artery-based flap: (**A**), nasolabial flap, with evidence of the facial artery as the pedicle; (**B**), retroangular flap, with evidence of angular artery as the pedicle, the grey shade indicates the subcutaneous tunneling; (**C**), island composite nasal flap, with exposure of the procerus muscle.

The *retroangular flap* (RAF) is a transpositional flap used in the reconstruction of the lower half of the nose, the lower eyelid, and the medial cheek. It is based on the angular artery, detected preoperatively by a Doppler. The flap is harvested from the nasolabial fold, with the first incision made in the distal part, to identify the angular pedicle. After isolating the vascular pedicle, the flap is islanded distal to medial with a subfascial dissection. After subcutaneous tunneling, the flap is inserted into the gap [10] (Figure 3B).

The *island composite nasal flap* (ic-NF) is adopted to increase the mobility of the distance covered by the classic nasolabial flap and is harvested using the procerus muscle near the defect as a pedicle. It is commonly used in the upper nasal region, the lower eyelid, and the medial canthal area. The flap is elevated under the muscle on the non-pedicle side and then advanced to the defect area. The donor site is closed with a V-Y technique. It can also be tunneled to reach more distant regions [10,16] (Figure 3C).

4. *Cervicofacial flap*: the cervicofacial flap is suited for moderate and large (>3 cm) defects of the cheek and is extendible to the periorbital and neck regions. It represents a combination of an advancement and rotational flap that can be moved anteriorly or posteriorly and anteriorly. The incision is a variant of the rhytidectomy approach but continues through the zygomatic arch, the lateral cantus, and the lower eyelid line until the nasolabial groove is reached in its most inferior part. The incision can be prolonged posteriorly, as in a parotidectomy with a horizontal limb. The flap is elevated superficially to the superficial musculoaponeurotic system (SMAS) and the masseteric fascia to avoid facial nerve branch injuries. After rotation and advancement, the donor site is closed by direct suture. Due to the great dimension of the flap, anchoring the flap to the orbital–zygomatic periosteum is necessary [11,17] (Figure 4).

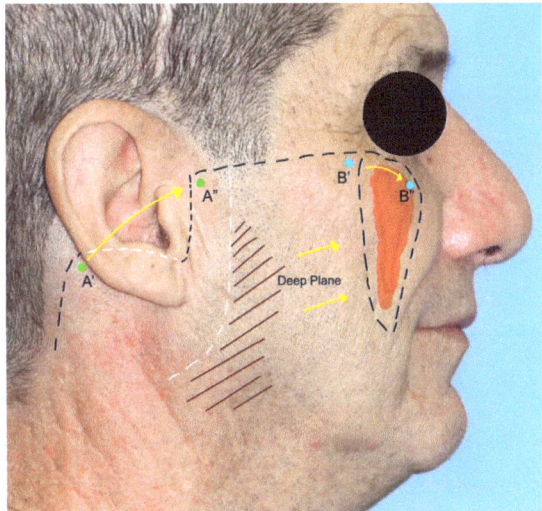

Figure 4. Cervicofacial flap. Part of the incision is hidden behind the ear lobe. During the dissection, a deep-plane incision is needed to permit the advancement of the flap. The skin has been marked with points A and B to show the incision's advancement.

5. *Paramedian forehead flap*: the paramedian forehead flap (PMFF) is an interpolated rotational flap harvested from the forehead and used for reconstructing large and complex defects of the nose. It is harvested based on the blood supply of the supratrochlear artery. The PMFF requires an accurate template of the defect to fill due to the complex three-dimensionality of the nasal region (Figure 4). After the identification of the supratrochlear pedicle by Doppler, the flap is harvested through the skin and subcutaneous muscle in a subfascial plan just above the periosteum. The key to the mobility of the flap is represented by the release of the corrugator muscle. The flap is rotated and then inset in the defect. The PMFF can be associated with cartilage grafting for composite reconstructions. In some variations of the technique, the pedicle is separated in a second stage debulking the flap excess [18] (Figure 5).

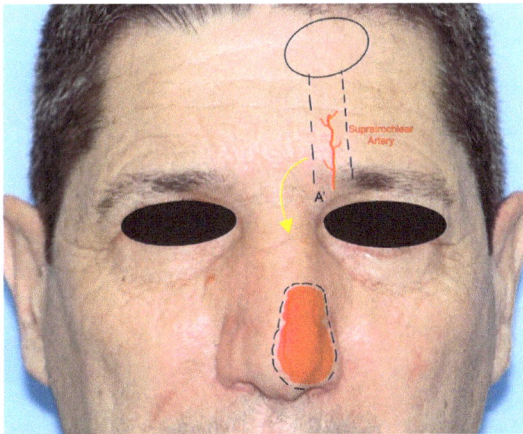

Figure 5. Paramedian forehead flap. The A' point represents the pivotal point for the flap rotation. The supratrochlear artery is shown as the pedicle of the flap.

6. *Frontal hairline island flap*: the frontal hairline island flap (FHiF) is a transpositional tunneled island flap harvested from the forehead and nourished by the supraorbital and supratrochlear arteries. It is used for medial canthal, upper nasal dorsum, and nasolabial small–medium defects. The FHiH is harvested in an elliptical shape at the level of the frontal hairline. Once the upper incision is made, the pedicle is dissected subperiosteally toward the orbital rim. The flap is transposed subcutaneously in a tunneled passage to the gap and sutured to the adjacent skin. The donor site is closed by direct suture. This flap represents a tunneled version of the paramedian flap but with indications for smaller skin defects [19] (Figure 6).

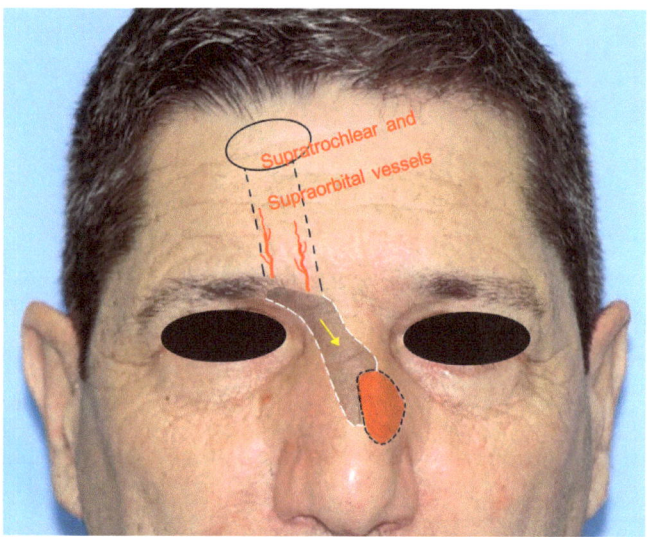

Figure 6. The frontal hairline island flap, with evidence of the vascular pedicle; the grey shade indicates the subcutaneous tunneling.

7. *Keystone flap*: the keystone area flap (KSAF) is a random-pattern multi-perforator advancement flap applicable to all defect dimensions, as it can be performed in all facial subunits. After tumor excision, the flap is islanded to the subcutaneous tissue with the shape of a Roman arch or vault keystone. The ratio between the width of the defect and the flap should be 1:1. The flap should not be undermined to not injure the multiple perforator vessels. It is important to preserve the superficial venous system and to keep intact the deep fascia. It is divided into four categories: type I is the classic keystone flap, type II includes skin grafting, type III is a double classic keystone, and type IV is based on undermining the skin around the keystone flap. The flap is then inserted into the gap and the closure starts with the edge closer to the defect. The longitudinal angles are closed in a V–Y fashion [8,20] (Figure 7).

8. *Karapandzic flap*: the Karapandzic flap (KF) is a rotation and advancement flap used in the upper lip and commissure reconstructions of full-thickness defects. It can fill medium and large defects. It is based on the facial artery branches. The KF is often harvested bilaterally with two "L-shaped" opposing flaps, eventually of different lengths. Once the upper lip skin defect has been created, a bull-horn skin excision is made in both alar sulci to increase the advancement of the flaps. The flap dissection is performed gently through the skin and subcutaneous tissue to preserve the vascular pedicle and the neural bundle. The two advancement flaps are moved until they meet centrally. Sutures are made by direct closure [21,22] (Figure 8).

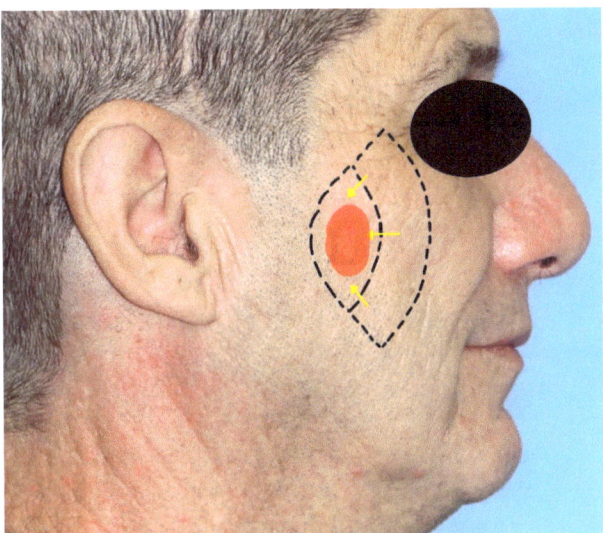

Figure 7. The keystone flap.

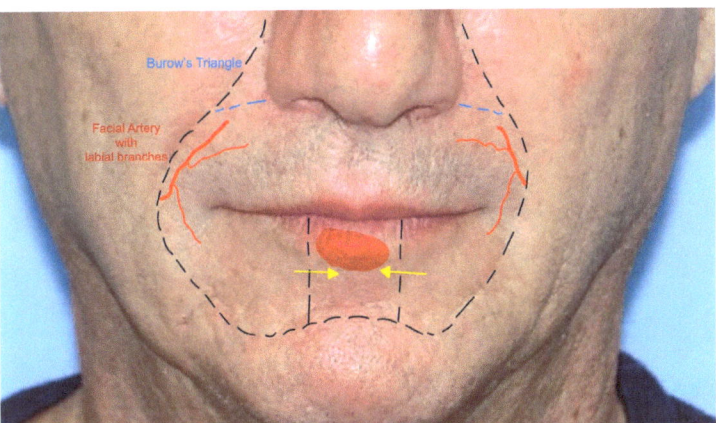

Figure 8. The Karapandzic flap: two Burow triangles are shown. The labial artery pedicle is indicated.

9. *Abbè flap*: the Abbè flap (AF) is a rotational flap usually harvested for the reconstruction of the upper lip. Its indications are defects involving 50% or more of the philtrum and defects of the medial element of the lateral subunit greater than 1.5 cm. The AF is considered a cross-lip switch flap, where the donor site is represented by a quadrangular full-thickness portion of the lower lip, frequently in its center–lateral part. The flap is based on the labial artery, the pedicle of the region, which can be medial or lateral in the flap harvested. The AF amount is calculated based on the defect to fill and then transposed with markers on the lower lip. Once the defect in the upper lip is created, the flap is rotated to fill the gap, while the lower lip is closed primarily. This technique temporarily reduces lip movement and mouth-opening due to the closure. The flap requires a second stage of division where the pedicle is cut and the flap is inserted. The flap can also be harvested for defects in the lower lip [23,24] (Figure 9).

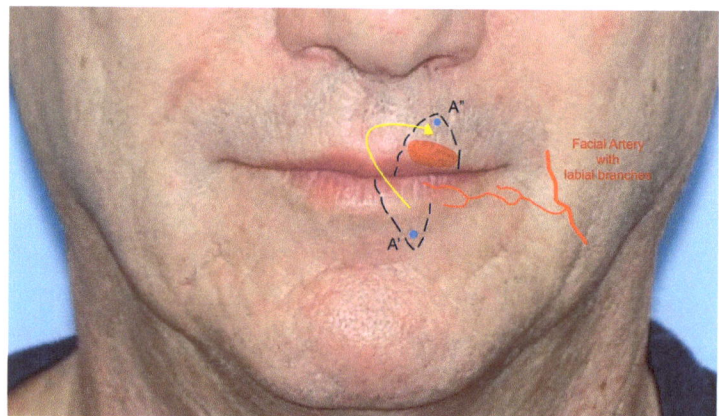

Figure 9. The Abbè flap: point A' is rotated and inserted in the upper lip, becoming point A". The branches of the labial artery are indicated.

10. *Mustardè flap*: the Mustardè flap is a rotational flap adopted for the reconstruction of large cheek defects, the lateral nose wall, and the lower eyelid region. Its harvesting begins from the edge of the excision defect and extends through the lower eyelid to the lateral canthus and ends with an incision superior and lateral to the temple region. The dissection is performed subcutaneously to not injure any facial nerve branches. As the MF is a flap of great dimensions, anchoring it to the zygomatic arch helps to avoid excessive tension on the flap's insertion. The donor site is closed by direct suture, with the help of Burow's triangles [25,26] (Figure 10).

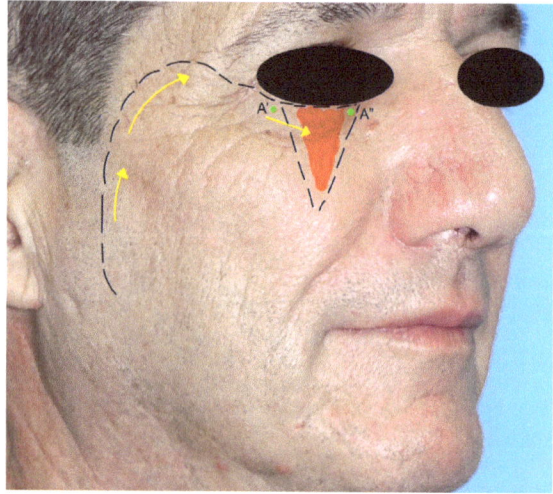

Figure 10. The Mustardè flap: the A' point is rotated to fill the skin gap till the A" point is reached.

4. Discussion

The reconstruction of facial defects after skin cancer excision can be challenging, especially in the midface, a region that requires both aesthetic and functional outcomes [23]. The division of the face into facial aesthetic subunits represents a valid method to delimitate the face into regions with their own characteristics and was first introduced by Gonzales-Ulloa in 1956 (Figure 11).

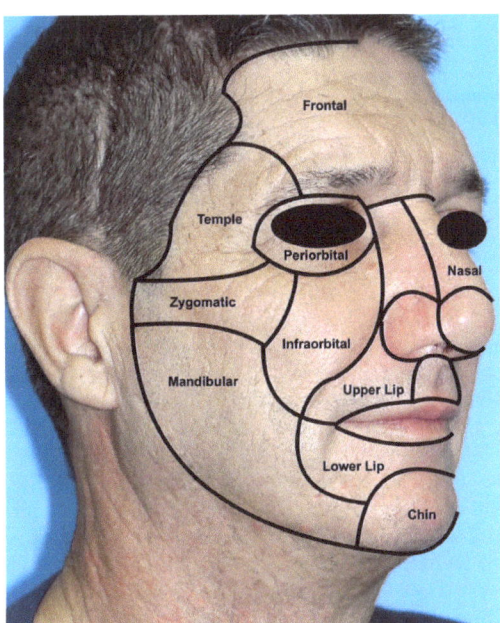

Figure 11. Gonzales-Ulloa aesthetic subunits of the face. From top to bottom: frontal, temple, periorbital, nasal, zygomatic, infraorbital, upper lip, lower lip, mandibular, and chin [4].

The utility of these subunits is double: on one hand, they delimitate areas with circumscribed histology, thickness, and texture; on the other hand, their separation lines represent marks for surgical incisions to keep areas with different characteristics separated [27]. When defect size and location permit, reconstruction should be carried out within the same subunit or using the most similar one to obtain an excellent texture and functional match [13]. The concept of subunits is the basis of all facial reconstructions, where the restoration must guarantee high results [28].

The gradual but significant evolution of reconstructive techniques has led to several solutions in the hand of a maxillofacial surgeon's repertoire [3]. The most adopted options are represented by skin grafts, locoregional flaps, and free flaps. Despite skin grafts being versatile, their aesthetic and functional outcomes are very poor. Free flaps are used for very large defects, require the expertise of microvascular surgery, and have longer operative times, which are not suitable for all patients. Pedunculated flaps, also called local or locoregional flaps, are more accessible to surgeons and considered more reliable in specific settings [6]. For these reasons, local flaps are considered the best reconstructive option for small to medium defects [7]. Local flaps are classified on the basis of the method of movement in advancement flaps, pivotal or rotational flaps, transposition flaps, and islanded flaps. Based on their blood supply, they can be divided into random, axial, and perforator flaps [29]. Depending on the distance between the flap and the gap to fill, the pedicle can be identified and moved within the subcutaneous tissue or skeletonized: the pedicle skeletonization increases vascular mobility and adds further degrees of rotation [3,16,17]. In the midfacial region, the main pedicle used is the facial artery and its branches, such as the angular artery, the labial arteries, and the dorsal nasal artery [16,30]. In particular defects, for example in the nasal region, flaps can derive from the forehead vascular plexus, where supratrochlear and supraorbital arteries are the main flap pedicles [18,31]. Doppler probe mapping of vascular pedicles is mandatory during midfacial reconstruction flap design as it allows for the individuation of precise vessel courses [14].

As shown in Table 1, the majority of midfacial flaps are dedicated to cheek and nose reconstruction, as they represent the most prominent areas of the face and, for this reason, are more exposed to traumatic injuries and ultraviolet damage [13,21]. The zygomatic–cheek region is burdened with the need to manage facial nerve branches, protected beneath the SMAS in most locations. A dissection in a plane superficial to that of the SMAS and the parotid–masseteric fascia represents a pillar of fundamental importance in the preparation of flaps in this region [16,29]. While the cheek area is flatter and composed of more similar subunits, the nasal region represents a very complex district. Nasal skin can be tricky during reconstruction: it is thick on the dorsum, tip, and alar region, but becomes thin in the upper dorsum, lateral walls, and columella [32]. Furthermore, the presence of geometrically complex subcutaneous structures such as nasal cartilage is considered a factor that increases the reconstructive difficulty [17]. In 2015, Chang et al. proposed an algorithm for the flap choice in midfacial defect reconstruction to simplify surgical planning. The algorithm was based on two variables: defects size bigger or smaller than 3 cm and their distance from the nasolabial fold. Defects larger than 3 cm require a perforator transposition flap without considering the distance from the nasolabial fold. Smaller defects distant from or just on the fold should be reconstructed with a V–Y advancement flap. Defects smaller than 3 cm and near the nasolabial fold should require a perforator-based transposition flap [15]. Comparing the algorithm with the results of a review of the literature conducted in this study, it is possible to assume that the trend is unchanged: the bigger the flap, the higher the need for a defined vascularization of the flap to guarantee optimal engraftment [33,34].

Locoregional flaps, while safe and reliable, are not without complications. The rate of complications is directly related to flap complexity and the dimension of the defect. Smaller and easier locoregional flaps are the most successful ones. The most common complications are the general ones such as edema, perioperative hemorrhage, hematomas, and infections. Due to the nature of pedunculated flaps, total flap loss is very rare. Partial flap necrosis can occur more often in rotational flaps for pedicle suffering: debridement resolves the issue and allows second-intention healing [9]. Technique complications are represented by pincushioning and standing cone deformities, more common in bilobed and rhombic flaps [10]. Specific regional complications are mostly associated with tension on flaps surrounding tissues, functional deformities, and donor site issues [8]. For example, the cervicofacial and Mustardè flaps, harvested close to the eyelid, are encumbered by the risk of ectropion and eye sagging [10,21]. Paramedian and forehead hairline island flaps are harvested for medium–large defects and their donor site wounds could require a split-thickness skin graft of a dermal substitute to be appropriately closed [18,35,36]. Nasal obstruction is a complication of nasal reconstruction and it is secondary to wound contraction, compromising internal and external nasal valves [31]. Labial flaps such as the Abbe and the Karapandzic flaps can cause functional impairments such as microstomia and lip incompetence to liquids, solvable with minor ancillary surgeries [19,20].

The authors described the most established and standardized techniques for the reconstruction of a complex area. Taking into account the potentially infinite imagination in the design of locoregional flaps, including all of them was conceptually unachievable. For these reasons, the technique selection considered mainstream flaps, not contemplating all possible technical variants and eventually derived techniques. Another limitation of the study concerns the adoption of only one international database as a technique source.

5. Conclusions

The midface is one of the most challenging regions to reconstruct for maxillofacial surgeons because of its dynamic functional and aesthetic components. The midfacial district has a complex structure that requires a detailed understanding of the facial subunits, the location and size of the defect, and the choice of the appropriate flap to achieve optimal outcomes. The reconstruction of the midfacial district with locoregional flaps involves a variety of surgical techniques. The use of these techniques requires a great emphasis on pre-surgical planning. In the conducted study, it was found that locoregional pedunculated flaps, due to their great variety, often represent the best solution for midfacial skin defects.

The success of the reconstruction of the midface using locoregional flaps depends on several key elements. One of the most critical elements is pre-surgical planning, which includes a detailed study of the facial subunits to identify the location, size, and extent of the defect. The surgeon must also consider the choice of the appropriate flap, which is crucial in achieving optimal outcomes. This should be carried out while paying attention to the vascular pedicles, which can make a significant difference in the success of the procedure.

In summary, the reconstruction of the midface using locoregional flaps is a complex procedure that requires a great emphasis on pre-surgical planning. Choosing the right flap, respecting the vascular pedicles, and understanding the facial subunits are key elements that determine the success of the procedure. Locoregional pedunculated flaps offer a great variety of options, making them often the best solution for midfacial skin defects.

Author Contributions: Conceptualization, G.S., C.C., F.M. (Fabio Maglitto), A.M., V.A., P.B. and A.S.; methodology, L.A.V., U.C. and A.M.; validation, G.S., C.C., A.M., P.B., L.C. and G.D.O.; formal analysis U.C.; investigation, L.A.V., U.C., F.M. (Fabio Maglitto), V.A., P.B. and A.S.; resources, F.M. (Francesco Maffia); data curation, F.M. (Francesco Maffia), F.M. (Fabio Maglitto), V.A. and A.S.; writing—original draft preparation, G.S., F.M. (Francesco Maffia) and L.A.V.; writing—review and editing, F.M. (Francesco Maffia); supervision, C.C., L.C. and G.D.O.; project administration, L.C. and G.D.O. All authors have read and agreed to the published version of the manuscript.

Funding: This research received no external funding.

Institutional Review Board Statement: Not applicable.

Informed Consent Statement: Written informed consent has been obtained from the patient to publish this paper.

Data Availability Statement: The data presented in this study are openly available in PubMed.

Acknowledgments: We are grateful to author Francesco Maffia for devoting himself to producing the graphical illustrations.

Conflicts of Interest: The authors declare no conflict of interest.

References

1. Rigby, M.H.; Hayden, R.E. Regional flaps: A move to simpler reconstructive options in the head and neck. *Curr. Opin. Otolaryngol. Head Neck Surg.* **2014**, *22*, 401–406. [CrossRef] [PubMed]
2. Ercan, A.; Ercan, L.D.; Demiroz, A. Nasolabial Perforator Flap: A Multi-Tool for Reconstruction of Facial Units. *J. Craniofac. Surg.* **2020**, *31*, 1042–1045. [CrossRef] [PubMed]
3. Hammer, D.; Vincent, A.G.; Williams, F.; Ducic, Y. Considerations in Free Flap Reconstruction of the Midface. *Facial Plast. Surg.* **2021**, *37*, 759–770. [CrossRef] [PubMed]
4. Gonzalez-Ulloa, M. Restoration of the Face Covering by Means of. *Br. J. Plast. Surg.* **1956**, *9*, 212–221. [CrossRef]
5. Nsaful, K.O. The Use of Rotation Flap to Cover a Facial Defect—A Case Study. *Mod. Plast. Surg.* **2020**, *10*, 101–107. [CrossRef]
6. Orabona, G.D.; Maffia, F.; Audino, G.; Abbate, V.; Germano, C.; Bonavolontà, P.; Romano, A.; Villari, R.; Mormile, M.; Califano, L. The Use of Matriderm® for Scalp Full-Thickness Defects Reconstruction: A Case Series. *J. Clin. Med.* **2022**, *11*, 6041. [CrossRef]
7. Gabrysz-Forget, F.; Tabet, P.; Rahal, A.; Bissada, E.; Christopoulos, A.; Ayad, T. Free versus pedicled flaps for reconstruction of head and neck cancer defects: A systematic review. *J. Otolaryngol. Head Neck Surg.* **2019**, *48*, 13. [CrossRef]
8. Yoon, C.S.; Kim, H.B.; Kim, Y.K.; Kim, H.; Kim, K.N. Relaxed skin tension line-oriented keystone-designed perforator island flaps considering the facial aesthetic unit concept for the coverage of small to moderate facial defects. *Medicine* **2019**, *98*, e14167. [CrossRef]
9. Lou, X.; Xue, C.; Molnar, J.A.; Bi, H. A Method to Reproduce Symmetry in Midfacial Reconstruction: A Report of 19 Cases. *Adv. Ski. Wound Care* **2020**, *33*, 383–388. [CrossRef]
10. Seo, Y.-J.; Hwang, C.; Choi, S.; Oh, S.-H. Midface Reconstruction with Various Flaps Based on the Angular Artery. *J. Oral Maxillofac. Surg.* **2009**, *67*, 1226–1233. [CrossRef]
11. Chu, E.A.; Byrne, P.J. Local Flaps I: Bilobed, Rhombic, and Cervicofacial. *Facial Plast. Surg. Clin. N. Am.* **2009**, *17*, 349–360. [CrossRef] [PubMed]
12. Durgun, M.; Özakpinar, H.R.; Sari, E.; Selçuk, C.T.; Seven, E.; Tellioğlu, A.T. The Versatile Facial Artery Perforator-Based Nasolabial Flap in Midface Reconstruction. *J. Craniofacial Surg.* **2015**, *26*, 1283–1286. [CrossRef] [PubMed]
13. Hon, H.H.; Chandra, S.R. Rhomboid Flap. *Atlas Oral Maxillofac. Surg. Clin.* **2020**, *28*, 17–22. [CrossRef] [PubMed]

14. Limberg, A.A. *Mathematical Principles of Local Plastic Procedures on the Surface of the Human Body*; Medgis: Leningrad, Russia, 1946.
15. Cook, T.A.; Israel, J.M.; Wang, T.D.; Murakami, C.S.; Brownrigg, P.J. Cervical rotation flaps for midface resurfacing. *Arch. Otolaryngol. Head Neck Surg.* **1991**, *117*, 77–82. [CrossRef]
16. Pepper, J.-P.; Baker, S.R. Local Flaps: Cheek and Lip Reconstruction. *JAMA Facial Plast. Surg.* **2013**, *15*, 374–382. [CrossRef]
17. Sakellariou, A.; Salama, A. The Use of Cervicofacial Flap in Maxillofacial Reconstruction. *Oral Maxillofac. Surg. Clin. N. Am.* **2014**, *26*, 389–400. [CrossRef]
18. Smart, R.J.; Yeoh, M.S.; Kim, D.D. Paramedian forehead flap. *Oral Maxillofac. Surg. Clin. N. Am.* **2014**, *26*, 401–410. [CrossRef]
19. Karsdağ, S.; Sacak, B.; Bayraktaroglu, S.; Özcan, A.; Ugurlu, K.; Bas, L. A novel approach for the reconstruction of medial canthal and nasal dorsal defects: Frontal hairline Island flap. *J. Craniofac. Surg.* **2008**, *19*, 1653–1657. [CrossRef]
20. Ettinger, K.S.; Fernandes, R.P.; Arce, K. Keystone Flap. *Atlas Oral Maxillofac. Surg. Clin.* **2019**, *28*, 29–42. [CrossRef]
21. Teemul, T.A.; Telfer, A.; Singh, R.P.; Telfer, M.R. The versatility of the Karapandzic flap: A review of 65 cases with patient-reported outcomes. *J. Cranio-Maxillofac. Surg.* **2016**, *45*, 325–329. [CrossRef]
22. Karapandzic, M. Reconstruction of lip defects by local arterial flaps. *Br. J. Plast. Surg.* **1974**, *27*, 93–97. [CrossRef] [PubMed]
23. Luce, E.A.; Jing, X.L.; Carlson, T. Abbe Flap Reconstruction of the Upper Lip. *Plast. Reconstr. Surg.* **2020**, *145*, 606e–607e. [CrossRef] [PubMed]
24. Quick, B. The Estlander-Abbe operation. *Aust N Z J. Surg.* **1946**, *16*, 142–148. [CrossRef]
25. Patel, S.B.; Buttars, B.R.; Roy, D.B. Mustardé flap for primary nasal sidewall defect post-Mohs micrographic surgery. *JAAD Case Rep.* **2022**, *23*, 151–154. [CrossRef] [PubMed]
26. Mustardé, J.C. The use of flaps in the orbital region. *Plast. Reconstr. Surg.* **1970**, *45*, 146–150. [CrossRef] [PubMed]
27. Chang, J.W.; Lim, J.H.; Lee, J.H. Reconstruction of midface defects using local flaps. *Medicine* **2019**, *98*, e18021. [CrossRef]
28. Neill, B.; Rickstrew, J.; Tolkachjov, S. Reconstructing the Glabella and Nasal Root. *J. Drugs Dermatol.* **2022**, *21*, 983–988. [CrossRef]
29. Vozel, D.; Stritar, A. Cheek reconstruction with vy, cervicofacial and submental flap. *Zdr. Vestn.* **2019**, *88*, 143–155.
30. Zhang, C.; Tang, X.; Wei, Z.; Wang, D.; Wang, B.; Zeng, X.; Jin, W. Nasolabial flap with Facial artery perforator for repairing defects after resection of midface tumor. *Zhonghua Zheng Xing Wai Ke Za Zhi = Chin. J. Plast. Surg.* **2016**, *32*, 342–346.
31. Zarrabi, S.; Welch, M.; Neary, J.; Kim, B.-J. A Novel Approach for Total Nasal Reconstruction. *J. Oral Maxillofac. Surg. Off. J. Am. Assoc. Oral Maxillofac. Surg.* **2019**, *77*, e1–e1073. [CrossRef]
32. Weber, S.M.; Baker, S.R. Management of Cutaneous Nasal Defects. *Facial Plast. Surg. Clin. N. Am.* **2009**, *17*, 395–417. [CrossRef] [PubMed]
33. Kim, S.W.; Kim, Y.H.; Kim, J.T. Angular artery perforator-based transposition flap for the reconstruction of midface defect. *Int. J. Dermatol.* **2012**, *51*, 1366–1370. [CrossRef] [PubMed]
34. Baker, S.R.; Swanson, N.A. Reconstruction of Midfacial Defects Following Surgical Management of Skin Cancer. *J. Dermatol. Surg. Oncol.* **1994**, *20*, 133–140. [CrossRef] [PubMed]
35. Zito, P.M.; Mazzoni, T. Paramedian Forehead Flaps. In *Stat Pearls [Internet]*; StatPearls Publishing: Treasure Island, FL, USA, 2022.
36. Petersen, W.; Rahmanian-Schwarz, A.; Werner, J.-O.; Schiefer, J.; Rothenberger, J.; Hübner, G.; Schaller, H.-E.; Held, M. The use of collagen-based matrices in the treatment of full-thickness wounds. *Burns* **2016**, *42*, 1257–1264. [CrossRef] [PubMed]

Disclaimer/Publisher's Note: The statements, opinions and data contained in all publications are solely those of the individual author(s) and contributor(s) and not of MDPI and/or the editor(s). MDPI and/or the editor(s) disclaim responsibility for any injury to people or property resulting from any ideas, methods, instructions or products referred to in the content.

MDPI AG
Grosspeteranlage 5
4052 Basel
Switzerland
Tel.: +41 61 683 77 34

Journal of Clinical Medicine Editorial Office
E-mail: jcm@mdpi.com
www.mdpi.com/journal/jcm

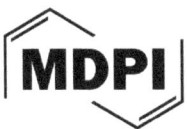

Disclaimer/Publisher's Note: The title and front matter of this reprint are at the discretion of the Guest Editor. The publisher is not responsible for their content or any associated concerns. The statements, opinions and data contained in all individual articles are solely those of the individual Editor and contributors and not of MDPI. MDPI disclaims responsibility for any injury to people or property resulting from any ideas, methods, instructions or products referred to in the content.

www.ingramcontent.com/pod-product-compliance
Lightning Source LLC
LaVergne TN
LVHW070002100526
838202LV00019B/2609